Mama Jude

Mama Jude

An Australian nurse's extraordinary other life in Africa

Judy Steel

with **Michael Sexton**

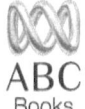
ABC Books

The ABC 'Wave' device is a trademark of the Australian Broadcasting Corporation and is used under licence by HarperCollins*Publishers* Australia.

First published in Australia in 2009
by HarperCollins*Publishers* Australia Pty Limited
ABN 36 009 913 517
harpercollins.com.au

Copyright © Judy Steel 2009

The right of Judy Steel to be identified as the author of this work has been asserted by her in accordance with the *Copyright Amendment (Moral Rights) Act 2000*.

This work is copyright. Apart from any use as permitted under the *Copyright Act 1968*, no part may be reproduced, copied, scanned, stored in a retrieval system, recorded, or transmitted, in any form or by any means, without the prior written permission of the publisher.

HarperCollins*Publishers*
25 Ryde Road, Pymble, Sydney, NSW 2073, Australia
31 View Road, Glenfield, Auckland 0627, New Zealand
A 53, Sector 57, Noida, UP, India
77–85 Fulham Palace Road, London W6 8JB, United Kingdom
2 Bloor Street East, 20th floor, Toronto, Ontario M4W 1A8, Canada
10 East 53rd Street, New York NY 10022, USA

National Library of Australia Cataloguing-in-Publication data:

Steel, Judy, 1943–
   Mama Jude : an Australian nurse's extraordinary other life in Africa / Judy Steel, Michael Sexton.
   1st ed.
   ISBN: 978 0 7333 2478 9 (pbk.)
   Steel, Judy, 1943-
   Nurses – Australia – Biography.
   Nurses – Uganda – Biography.
   Medical care – Uganda.
   Uganda – Social conditions.
   Sexton, Michael (Michael Dean), 1964-
610.73092

Cover design by Peter Long
All photos courtesy Judy Steel and UACO
Typeset in 11/18pt LT Garamond Light by Kirby Jones

To Allan, the love of my life, for his love and strength

To Fiona, David and Peter, for understanding that their mother did something different

For Michael, Joshua, Timothy, Zachary, Cameron, Claire, John and Kate, so that one day they will understand why Nanna went to Africa

*Progress of the soul consists
not in thinking much,
but in loving much.*
St Teresa of Avila

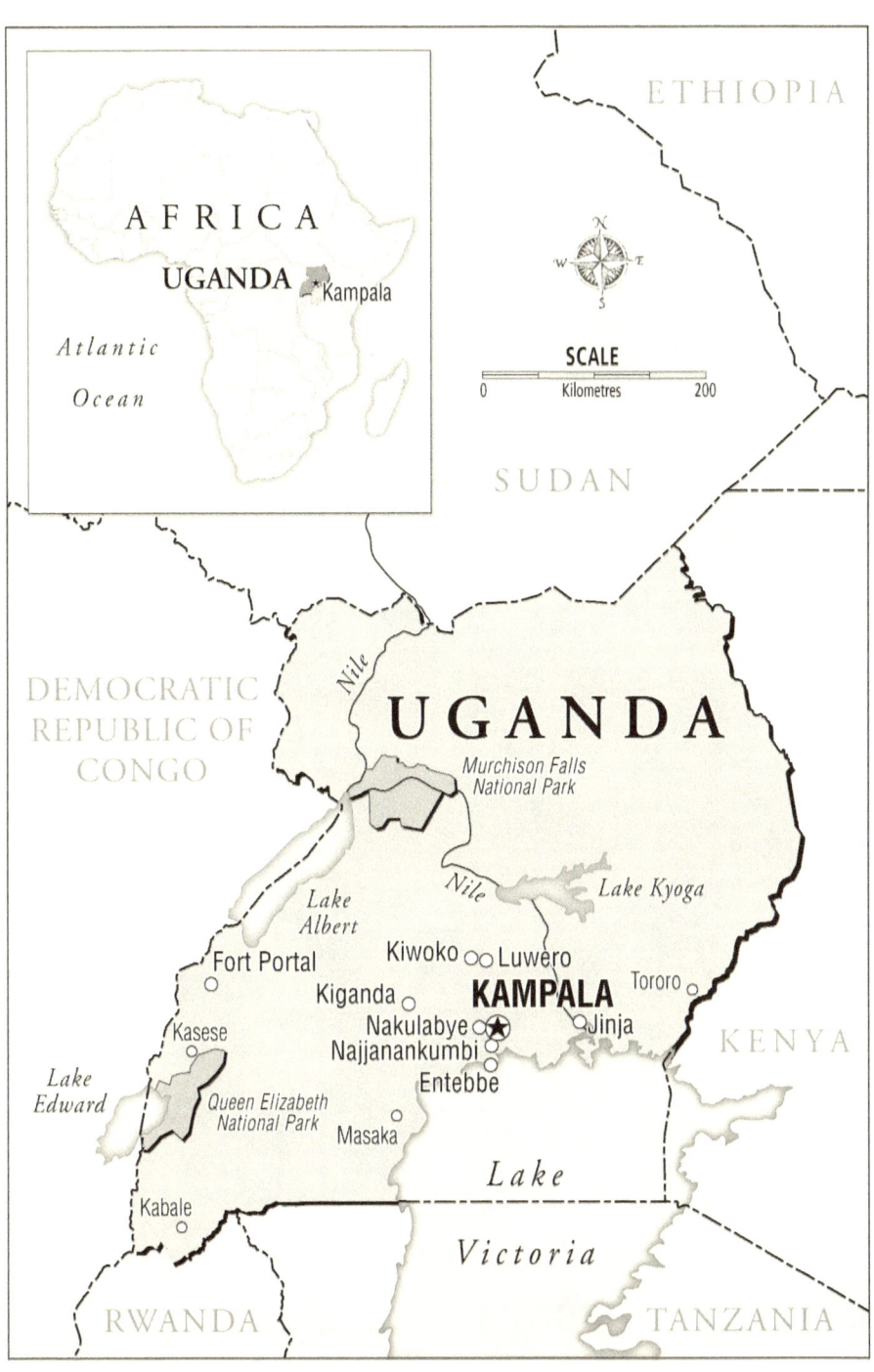

Prologue

UGANDA IS A COUNTRY where there is much love and much beauty. It is a place where people laugh and dance, broad smiles lighting up black faces. When they dance, Ugandan women ululate in a high pitch, swaying their shoulders and arms while rolling their often ample hips. They love bright clothes that catch the light and complement their rhythm. Mostly dancing takes place outdoors and the foot stomping sends clouds of dust into the air that settles as streaks of mud on sweaty faces and arms. It is an outpouring of an internal joy and can go on for hours. It doesn't have to be a wedding, but this is where I found myself amongst such exuberance in mid 2008.

It is the end of my seventh visit to Uganda and, as usual, I am physically and emotionally exhausted. I think back to my first trip almost a decade previously, when I arrived knowing virtually nothing of this extraordinary country. All I'd hoped was to be able to help its people in some way before returning to my 'normal' life. At fifty-six years old and at the end of a successful career as a nurse and administrator, my husband, Allan, and I should have been planning our retirement travels and spending time with our growing number of grandchildren, but instead I had stepped off a plane at Entebbe on the edge of Lake Victoria, a forty five-minute drive from Uganda's capital, Kampala.

Over the next three months on that first trip, and then during another three months the following year, I saw things that almost broke my spirit. Parts of Uganda are places of deep despair, where serious illness is so common that people expect to die young simply because that is what happens to almost everyone they know or see. When HIV/AIDS spread across the globe, it took deep root in sub-Saharan Africa. Generations have been stripped away leaving the very old caring for the very young, while HIV-positive mothers pass the infection to their babies while still in the womb. Drugs that extend life and ease the pain of HIV in other parts of the world have been unavailable or outrageously expensive in Uganda. When visiting men and women in the agonising final stages of the disease, I could offer almost nothing other than some dignity in death.

Pauline has AIDS and so does her new husband, Johnson, but this does not stop them dancing at their wedding reception, held in the grounds of the Busabala Road Hospital in Najjanankumbi, a slum area on the edges of Kampala. This is where I first found renewal amid the death and despair all those years ago.

The hospital was built by the most committed doctor I have ever met, Edward Ssembatya. Out of his own money he had bought the land, paid for the materials and, brick by brick, seen a hospital grow. When we first met in 1999, his generosity had stretched his resources so far that it seemed to me that it would take a miracle to complete the facility he dreamt of. But his commitment inspired me to start a charity which, with the backing of generous Australians, would one day see the hospital complete and filled with beds and equipment. After two visits to Uganda, I returned in 2001 to oversee the delivery of a shipping container packed with donated hospital equipment and medical supplies we had collected in Australia. After being emptied, the container was fashioned into a primary health care clinic in the grounds of Edward's hospital. Two years later we had collected enough equipment to send a second container. The size of the clinic doubled and a rehabilitation centre for physiotherapy was created.

It wasn't long before a vibrant youth movement and a support group for those with HIV/AIDS evolved from these facilities. Widows who have lost husbands to the disease also meet twice a month to socialise and support others in the community, while the clinic provides free immunisation for 7000 children per year and hosts classes to teach the mamas good health practices.

Micro-loans were the next phase in this remarkable community transformation, and AIDS widows now run cafés, pig farms and an alterations shop to create income streams. To help others qualify for loans there is now an adult literacy school with a growing waiting list. Edward's initial dream of a hospital for the poor is moving toward a self-sustaining community that is attracting keen interest from across the country.

Pauline, our bride today, is one of those studying to read and write. When she started literacy classes I asked her what her goal was; she replied that she simply wanted the dignity of being able to write her own name before she died. With the help of treatment and improved diet, that ambition has grown and she has now taken out a small loan to start a business selling charcoal. Now this beautiful young woman stands before me in her wedding dress.

After the ceremony, Pauline changes into a long, sparkly red dress. Still wearing her tiara and glittery earrings, she looks stunning as I stand in line to present a gift. When my turn comes she starts to dance towards me, and so I dance towards her. There is a huge roar from the crowd and many jump to their feet. We dance and laugh and hug. In this beautiful, precious, terminally ill woman is Uganda.

I didn't expect to see any of this but I have. This country has shown me the heights and depths of humanity and tested me in a way I could never imagine. Although I have cried an ocean of tears and sat helplessly watching people waste and die, Uganda has shown me much about loving and caring, about resilience and renewal. Should I sit on the dirt floor of a sweltering shack in despair because another person has succumbed to AIDS, or can something be done?

How I came to be in Uganda at all is a story that evolves from a child in India and a flash flood in the Australian outback. My name is Judy Steel and in Uganda I am a *mzungu*, or white person, but they call me Mama Jude.

Chapter One

I USUALLY SAY THAT the preparation for my work in Africa began in the final years of my working life in Adelaide, but it probably really started when I was a child growing up in the tiny country town of Nangwarry in the south-east of South Australia. The region has good rainfall and was the first area of Australia to begin commercial forestry after pine plantations were established in the 1870s. After a timber mill was built in 1939, the town quickly expanded as houses sprang up for the growing number of timber workers and their families.

We moved to Nangwarry in 1947, when I was four. I had been very sick with pneumonia and, on the doctor's advice, Mum and Dad got me out of the city. While a medical condition was the reason for leaving, it was also the reason we were in Adelaide in the first place. My parents met at Calvary Hospital where my father, Laurie McIver, had been admitted to have his appendix out. There he met a nurse named Lenore McCarthy. In those days you couldn't be engaged and work at Calvary, so Mum moved to Blackwood Hospital in the Adelaide Hills until they were married.

The day we left Adelaide was one of those summer scorchers and the stuffy car was made all the worse by having three kids crammed in alongside our possessions. The car had curtains fitted instead of glass windows, and I kept losing handkerchiefs out of the little window. We ran out of petrol before getting to Naracoorte and Dad had to hitch a ride to find more. During the wait I managed to cut my toe, so Mum had to find a bandage in all of the packed things.

Despite this difficult beginning, life in Nangwarry was wonderful. Our childhood was safe and we knew everyone in the town. Dad had been a metal worker at the Islington Railway Yards in Adelaide and had no problem finding work at the sawmill. Us kids all played together, often in a big pine tree in the next street from us; every night in summer after tea we would congregate to climb it. Most of the boys would hang around the bottom to try to look up our skirts. We would go on bike rides together and, if we didn't have enough, the boys would ride and the girls would sit on the handlebars and steer. One day we were a few miles up the road toward Penola when we had a pile-up. I was on the bottom and finished up with a badly cut and infected knee. Mum had to drive me to Mount Gambier many times for penicillin injections while Dad made me a cradle out of pine to keep the blankets off it while I was in bed.

When the mill was closed we would climb up the huge hill of sawdust at the back and slide down on a piece of tin. In summer we would go into the pine forest with a bottle of cordial and some biscuits. There was a pond off the Kalangadoo road and we would tie a string around the bottle and drop it in the water to cool it down and then have a picnic when we had finished playing. We were quite wicked when the city cousins came to visit, taking them out to the pines and then hiding from them. In hindsight it was a terrible thing to do.

My older sister, Elaine, and younger brother, Bob, always seemed a lot smarter than me and did well at school. I don't remember ever coming first but I did alright. When we were still in primary school, Mum contracted polio so Elaine and I went to live with our grandmother, Catherine McCarthy, in Jamestown. She was our only living grandparent and we developed a loving relationship with her. She was tall, had a wonderful sense of humour and taught us how to make pavlova.

After Mum recovered she had to learn to walk again. When we came home from Jamestown, she staggered from chair to chair in the kitchen, retraining her limbs. Dad bought a fridge so she didn't have to bother with the ice chest. Despite this, she always seemed to be happy and smiling and had the love of beautiful friends in Nangwarry.

In later years a stroke left Grandma paralysed down one side and unable to speak. She came to live with us and slept in my room, and I looked after her during the night if she needed to go to the toilet. This was when I really got to know and love my grandmother. She would play cards managing with one hand and I remember her laughing a lot. I never saw her angry or upset about her lot in life. She died when I was fifteen, and in hindsight this time with her taught me about accepting the good with the bad.

We were Catholic and along with the Mount Gambier parish priest, Dad and a few of his friends just about built the church at Nangwarry themselves. The building, which was across the road from our house, was used as a school during the week and a church on Sunday. I spent all my primary school years there being taught by the St Joseph nuns. The order was founded in south-eastern South Australia by Mary MacKillop, who came to nearby Penola in 1859 to help the local priest, Father Julian Tenison Woods, establish a school. They decided to start an order of women dedicated to serving the poor in remote country areas and their school in Penola was opened in 1866. Mary moved on to Adelaide and later Sydney, where the Josephite order became known for its work with schools, orphanages and refuges for women and the elderly.

The nuns lived in the house next door and became an integral part of our life. There was a little gate between our properties where we would slip in and out, because Mum and Dad were always doing something for them. During the holidays, Mum would drive the nuns in our car and take them on picnics. The nuns taught me to play the piano at the convent, though I wish I had learnt to sing as well. Mum played the piano and Dad would accompany her with his lovely, strong tenor voice; the love of music and singing which they instilled in me have been integral parts of my life. I still sing in the church choir and am learning the violin.

My secondary schooling was at the Josephite convent in Penola. I left during my intermediate year (year 10) to take up a clerical position with the Penola council. A short time later I took a position forty kilometres away in Mount Gambier where my sister, Elaine, was working. We boarded in Mount Gambier during the week and came home on weekends. This was a wonderful time in our lives, with boyfriends and weekly dances at Tarpeena or Mount Gambier. On my sixteenth birthday, Mum, Dad and my brother shifted to Mount Gambier where they bought their first house, so we were all able to live together once more. That same year I made my debut, along with all the other young women in the south-east. Debuts were very popular then and many churches and other organisations had their own balls. There was the Debutante of the Year ball at the end of the season, when all the local girls and their partners were invited to attend a huge function at the Mount Gambier Show Hall.

While still working at the mill my father became ill with multiple sclerosis, which developed into an inflammation of the spinal cord known as transverse myelitis. He became very disabled and Mum nursed him for twenty-seven years before he finally died on St Patrick's Day in 1978, aged sixty-eight. He was a beautiful human being and never once did I hear him complain as he battled the disease, eventually becoming bed-bound. When he died we were all around him, and my mother's last words to him were 'Goodbye, darling'. I don't know how Mum did everything that she did for him, and never once did I hear her complain either. Through their actions they taught me a lesson in unconditional love. After Dad died, Mum continued living in Mount Gambier and I would travel from Adelaide to spend a week with her every few months. We would shop, go out for meals and have a 'happy hour' before dinner each evening. Often Elaine would join us for lots of girl time and plenty of laughs.

Shortly after making my debut, I began to like the idea of nursing. I was accepted at Mount Gambier Hospital to commence training but changed my mind and went instead to the Royal Adelaide Hospital, which was the main teaching hospital in South Australia. On 17 July 1961, I started out as a very green young trainee nurse who had no idea what constituted a blood vessel, that the stomach was an organ, or even what the body looked like. Some of the girls had studied science and biology and were streets ahead of me. But what I did know was how to care about a fellow human being, and I quickly fitted into Preliminary Training School (PTS) at Ayres House opposite the Royal Adelaide, which is now an elegant restaurant. We slept in the nurses' home 'three to a room' and some of the nurses I met, such as Pam Henwood from Barmera on the River Murray, became lifelong friends.

PTS lasted six weeks, after which I was sent to Verco Ward, the first stop on my three-year training journey to become a registered nurse. Verco was a men's medical ward built pre-war as a temporary building, but was still in use thirty years later. We worked six days a week and never finished our shifts on time. I still have the happiest and saddest memories of this period. I saw my first dead person; sometimes there were three deaths in a day. I learnt that male patients like to play jokes on green nurses, almost all of which are best not repeated. I learnt how to scrub bedpans and urinals and how to wash and powder gloves ready for sterilisation in the autoclave.

My favourite period was the six months I spent in casualty (now called accident and emergency), which was all about thinking on your feet and responding to every kind of emergency. The only thing that ever turned my stomach was when a lady came in one Sunday afternoon after her big toe had an altercation with a lawnmower.

During my third year I worked in the operating theatre for six months, often hard going with some operations lasting up to twelve hours. The most challenging was the night shift over Easter, when many accident victims needed emergency surgery. My previous experience in casualty had taught me to react quickly in emergencies. I had fabulous teachers at the Royal Adelaide, both in the classroom and the ward. At the same time, there were a few renowned for making life difficult no matter how hard you worked. Rita Huppatz was matron most of my time at the Royal, a beautiful, gentle woman who could make you feel so special, but if you had done something wrong you would wish the floor would open up and swallow you – like when she found me sitting on the bed of an ill nurse who I had gone to visit in the sick bay. I learnt quickly that you didn't have to raise your voice to get your point across. In fact, it was far more effective if you spoke quietly.

It was during my second year on night duty in casualty that I met the man who I was to share my life with. In hindsight I smile to myself remembering that my parents had also met in a hospital. It was a quiet night and I was busying myself in the steriliser room, placing instruments into the autoclave. I heard a noise at the door and looked up to see a handsome St John Ambulance driver watching me. Tall, with clear blue eyes, a ready smile and an obvious love of life and helping others, he had brought a patient in and was enjoying the warmth of the hospital. I thought he was probably after a cup of coffee as it was 3 am and cold outside. We got talking and I remembered seeing him several times during the previous few weeks when he and his attendant had brought other injured and sick people into casualty. Night shift was part of my job, but he had a day job and worked as a St John volunteer at night. We talked easily and this led to many more early morning assignations in casualty over a cup of coffee. I wonder in hindsight if Allan did all those night duties solely out of concern for the suffering or if he had an ulterior motive. One night he said to me, 'Would you go out with a policeman?' I replied, 'I've never been asked.' It transpired that Allan had been accepted as a police recruit and was about to commence his training. Of course I said yes, and our courtship commenced.

Allan had grown up in Adelaide as the middle child of Nell and John Steel. Before we met he had been a cabinet-maker and worked for a period in petrol stations servicing cars and later selling tyres and farm machinery. After joining the South Australia Police Department, as it was then called, he served for thirty-four years before retiring with the rank of chief superintendent. In 1986 he was one of the first recipients of the

Australian Police Medal and in later years he was also awarded the Police Service Medal.

At the end of three fabulous, tiring, hardworking and memorable years at the Royal Adelaide Hospital I became a registered nurse. Allan and I married as soon as we could after my training finished in January 1965. It was another of those awfully hot Adelaide days, and our friends and relatives had travelled from around South Australia to share it with us. Our honeymoon was spent in a borrowed caravan touring South Australia and Victoria. When we returned we were off again, moving about three hours north of Adelaide to Port Augusta, where Allan had been posted.

Port Augusta is often referred to as the crossroads of Australia because it is where the railway intersects north–south from Alice Springs to Adelaide and east–west from Sydney to Perth. The town had plenty of heavy industry with the railways, the port and a coal-fired power station that generated much of the state's electricity. Despite sitting on the Spencer Gulf, it can be unbearably hot in summer, with furnace-hot northerly winds sweeping off the inland deserts bringing clouds of stinging dust. Once when my parents came to visit, a horrific dust storm blew up while I collected them from the railway station. I had set the table for lunch and, on our return, had to empty the sand out of the spoons on the table.

The forty-plus temperatures coupled with a lack of trees didn't make a great impression on me; neither Allan nor I had ever experienced this kind of heat before. I remember there were oleanders everywhere and I have never liked them since.

The good news was that our little house was on the front street of the suburb of Willsden, which overlooked the Gulf, so we were always first to get the cool change.

In no time at all I was working at the hospital and about one week later was pregnant. David was born in December 1965, Peter came along two years later and Fiona was born in July 1970.

I learnt to be very resourceful after the babies arrived. We couldn't afford to buy a fan so I would soak bath towels in water and clip them over open windows so any breeze would evaporate the water and, in doing so, cool the house. We also draped wet towels over the clothes horse and then placed the baby near it. It was my early version of air conditioning.

In between having babies I worked part-time at the hospital, mostly on night duty where I used all my training in casualty and theatre. There were frequent road crashes, assaults and general emergency situations. In those days there was no flying doctor staff, so once I flew up to the opal-mining town of Andamooka to do a retrieval. Sometimes we would have to do a dash to Adelaide with a critically sick person and we all had enduring friendships with the ambulance staff in Port Augusta. Allan continued his volunteer ambulance work at night when I was home with the children.

It wasn't always easy living in Port Augusta, particularly being married to a policeman, but we were young and strong and we coped. We didn't have a phone or a second car, so to get David to kindergarten I would walk a mile and back twice a day while pushing a pram and carrying a toddler.

After seven years living in the 'Iron Triangle', as the area is commonly known, we moved to Salisbury in Adelaide's northern suburbs where Allan was the police prosecutor at the Elizabeth Magistrates Court. A year later he was moved to the city and we found ourselves living in an old police station on South Road at Edwardstown. This is the main south–north corridor through Adelaide, so trucks, semi-trailers and emergency vehicles thundered past day and night. The sirens especially seemed to be non-stop.

Even our three-year-old, Fiona, said we were suffering from noise pollution. In addition to the din, it was dangerous crossing to catch the school bus with two little boys. Although I had spent many holidays on farms, Allan's relatives were all in the city and he had long wanted to live on the land. So we took the plunge and bought a twenty-hectare farm in the Adelaide Hills near Nairne, about an hour's drive out of the city. Allan continued working in town, commuting each day.

This was the beginning of five years of hard work and a love affair with country life. One of my loveliest memories is of milking our house cow before the children woke up, watching the Murray River light up like a silver streak with the light of dawn before the first planes took off from Adelaide and flew overhead. The farm already had an intensive piggery and we were on a vertical learning curve as far as breeding them went, plus we had a small herd of cows bred for beef. Allan and I spent many a night dozing on a bale of hay in the piggery when we had a sow due to farrow.

Once Allan spent a week in hospital having his appendix removed and, as luck would have it, one of the sows farrowed at the same time. Twelve-year-old David learnt very quickly how to hold the piglets by one leg while I injected them with iron, while Allan's job of removing their needle teeth with electrician's side cutters (so they wouldn't bite each other and mum) also fell to me. In addition to the farm work, Allan continued full-time with the police while I worked as a weekend supervisor at Adelaide's Memorial Hospital.

As he grew older, David decided he wanted a career in the air force while Peter was seriously thinking of enlisting in the army. We decided to sell the farm and move back to Belair in the Adelaide Hills closer to the city, so they could join the air and army cadets to gauge if this was the life they wanted. It wasn't a tough decision because we wanted to do the best for them, but Allan still yearns for his Ferguson TEA 20 tractor and a few hectares of land to drive it on.

Both boys joined up the minute they finished their schooling, David into the RAAF and Peter into the Australian Army. David became a pilot and flew Hercules aircraft until eventually joining Qantas. Peter also became a pilot flying Blackhawk helicopters. Not to be outdone, Fiona followed her brother into the air force a few years later. I have always felt we missed out on something with the children choosing the careers they did. Of course, many of my friends also said we were spared the worry of them staying out all night, but I felt their absence greatly and had to learn how to say goodbye without making a complete ass of myself. Over the years I have continued to feel jealous of friends whose children and grandchildren are nearby. I think I always will.

We had not been back in Adelaide long when my father died. After watching Dad suffer and fight his transverse myelitis for so many years, including in the latter stages when his legs became gangrenous, I found I'd had enough of hospitals and doctors and needed some time away from nursing. I helped out waitressing for my aunt and uncle who ran a catering business.

But before long I found myself working at the Kalyra Hospital in the foothills south of Adelaide where I spent five years in the rehabilitation and hospice wards before there was a major turning point in my life. With the encouragement of the director of nursing, Jill Ashby, I applied to study part-time at university and was accepted, a remarkable turn of events to me seeing as I had not even completed year 10 at high school. I was terrified for about two weeks and kept asking myself what I was doing there when everyone else seemed to know so much more than me. However, as I've always done, I hung in there – and studied, studied, studied. My family were understanding and would often suggest I go to our holiday shack at Port Elliot for the weekend to finish a paper. In two years I earned a diploma in applied science/nursing management.

With new qualifications, I successfully applied for the position of matron at the Mitcham Resthaven Home for the Aged in 1985. A not-for-profit community service of the Uniting Church, Resthaven was one of the largest aged care organisations in

South Australia with nine sites and over a thousand residents. At the time, the Mitcham site had over a hundred residents in nursing home and hostel accommodation.

I felt that my new role as a matron would be best served if I added to my university education, so enrolled for a Bachelor of Nursing, which I completed in 1987. Resthaven gave me permission to attend lectures twice a week and I fulfilled any extra management duties with Resthaven after hours. It was a huge year, but worth it. My secretary, Anne Joyce, had been at Resthaven Mitcham for years and knew all the residents and their relatives. She protected me when I needed protecting and taught me about the intricacies of the place – we became lifelong friends.

During this time the Federal government introduced badly needed standards to improve the quality of life in nursing homes, and I had not been at Resthaven long when the nursing home was rebuilt. Everyone, including the residents, was involved in the planning, and I really enjoyed the interaction with builders, interior designers and Resthaven executive management. During construction there were peepholes in the temporary walls so residents could watch the men at work (and tell them where they were going wrong). At the end we had a fabulous party to celebrate.

After eight years at Mitcham I felt the need for a fresh challenge and found it in a newly created position at head office as director of care. It was a challenge to be in charge of people who had been my peers but also a great opportunity to develop what became a successful continence management policy.

For some time, financial reports and budgets had suggested too much money was being spent on laundry because of an inadequate approach to urinary incontinence in the frail aged. I felt very strongly that people had the right to a better quality of life and not to suffer such an anti-social and dehumanising condition. Historically, people in nursing homes with incontinence were simply changed out of their wet clothes at certain times. In consultation with others, I developed a program of care that enabled the sufferer to be toileted at a time convenient to them (instead of the staff) and as a result many of them then became dry. Changing the behaviour of nurses also improved the outlook for many residents: some renewed relationships with their families and went on outings because they were no longer embarrassed.

Resthaven became known for this new way of caring and I was asked to present papers and write articles for national and international publications. I have always been proud of this accomplishment; it didn't come naturally to me but, in my mind, the girl who did not complete year 10 kept returning to remind me that if you want to do something badly enough and you work hard enough, you can achieve it.

In 1997 Allan and I fulfilled some travel dreams. We flew to England via Africa as one of our aims was to see Victoria Falls in Zimbabwe, and it was while we stood at the top of the falls that I remarked that you couldn't look at this and not believe in God.

On reflection, it was a surprising thing to say because I was not overly religious. I had been brought up in a Christian home, given a Christian education and wonderful examples of Christian life from my parents, but I was not a frequent churchgoer.

After travelling through Europe, we headed home via India. Allan's mother had lived in Jabalpur until she was seventeen while her father was employed by Indian Railways. She had often spoken about her life there and, in particular, the Taj Mahal. We spent five days travelling in a car with a guide, seeing just a small part of the magic, mystique and wretchedness that is India. But it was while we were driving from Agra to Jaipur that something happened which I believe was the starting point of the rest of my life.

Stopped at a state border to pay a tax, Allan and I were alone in the car when a little girl, about ten years old, came up to my window. She carried her baby brother, perhaps ten months old, who was naked except for a piece of string around his waist. The girl's yellow and brown dress was clean, but the fastener was broken. In all of my life the people I knew could afford clothes, food and shelter. I was shattered that this baby boy was naked and the girl had only her dress on and they both were hungry.

The girl knocked on my car window and then put her fingers into her mouth, indicating food. We had been warned not to give beggars anything as it could start a riot, but a refusal felt beyond me here and tears welled up in my eyes. I said to Allan that I just had to give this child something. Our hotel had packed us a picnic breakfast because we had left very early, so Allan suggested we give her some food. I rolled down the window and handed her some food, which was wrapped in foil and was still warm. She very gently set her little brother down and, unwrapping the parcel, fed him three tiny morsels, taking nothing for herself. She then wrapped up the parcel, picked up her little brother and slowly walked away, presumably taking it home to share with her family. My last memory is of her looking back at me and smiling. I remember saying to Allan, 'I think that I have just been taught a very important lesson.' Here I was on the three-month trip of a lifetime wanting for nothing and yet a tiny beggar was so gracious, giving only to her brother and going without herself.

Sometimes I wish I had taken her photo, and yet that would have been an intrusion. I don't really need the printed image because, all these years later, I still see her vividly in my mind.

Chapter Two

I RETURNED TO WORK feeling restless and humbled. The only thing I was sure of was that, after thirty-seven years of nursing, I would be retiring sooner rather than later. With Allan already retired, I was being spoiled with my live-in housekeeper taking care of me, doing the shopping and generally making life easy. But whenever I least expected it, a little voice inside my head was repeating, 'You've had a wonderful life – it's time to give something back.' But, after working in an aged care organisation for so many years, I felt that I didn't want to become involved in volunteering in that sort of environment. I remember saying to friends that when I retired I was definitely *not* going to be a volunteer. I wanted to learn smocking, read books, play with my grandchildren and cook.

In April 1997, Allan and I set off to visit our son Peter and daughter-in-law Katrina in Townsville. We drove through the outback in our four-wheel-drive, off-road camper trailer in tow, following a stock route about a hundred kilometres north-east of Innamincka close to the South Australia–Queensland border. Having checked that the weather forecast was good, we made camp for the night. The next morning, it started pouring just after seven and forty-five minutes later we'd had fifty millimetres of rain. By the end of the day we'd had three times that and were marooned. Although we had a phone, UHF radio and car radio, we couldn't receive anything.

We spent four days and nights mostly in our car. Allan read every page of the Pajero manual and played patience balancing cards on the back of a satchel. I knitted a jumper for my grandson. We slept the first two nights in the front of the car and it was freezing. It was impossible to get the trailer open because it was covered in mud which had set like a rock. Every time Allan got out to check the creek level he would grow several centimetres taller with the thick, tenacious mud on his boots. If we tried to drive the car we slipped around with no traction at all; it was terrifying. We had plenty of food and water but couldn't heat anything for the first two days. On the third day we were able to prise open the trailer and cook food on the gas stove but were still unable to move. I could almost hear the radio station reports: 'Fears are held for the safety of a middle-aged couple travelling in the outback ...' I imagined our two sons, both pilots, beside themselves searching for their parents.

There was nothing we could do but wait. Then something strange happened, which I later came to call 'The Challenge'. At 4.45 pm on the second day, the sky became pitch black while the baked red earth of the outback turned a brilliant gold. I was alone as Allan was out walking about half a kilometre away, checking a stock tank to see if we could replenish our water supplies. I was so overawed by this landscape that I snapped a photograph, which I have since called my postcard from heaven. Over the years I had never stopped loving God but had stopped going to church. But in the past few months we had started going to Westbourne Park Uniting Church because I wanted a spiritual life similar to the example of my parents. Sitting alone in the car amid breathtaking scenery my emotions turned from awe to anger. I felt marooned, isolated and very frightened. This was supposed to be a holiday to see our son and family and I didn't want to be stuck in the mud. Inexplicably I suddenly started sobbing, crying out to God, 'What do you want from me?'

I had been terrified that we would be inundated with more rain and be marooned for weeks, but not one more drop of rain fell. The next day I was sitting in the car looking around at the drenched landscape when I had a strange vision of myself holding a black baby and surrounded by black children. I had no idea where these children were from, apart from a strong feeling that it was somewhere in Africa.

After three days we were finally able to get the camper trailer opened and things started drying out. By the end of the week we were travelling north in the hope of getting closer to civilisation. We had gone about fifteen kilometres when we came to a very long patch of mud and became bogged up to our axles. After inspecting the problem, Allan declared it could not be worse and we couldn't get out. With this I just cried and asked Allan, 'Haven't I been tested enough?' Allan told me everything would work out okay and, no surprises, it did. Although the nearest town was still hundreds of kilometres away, we were close enough to be heard on our UHF radio and, within half an hour of our emergency call, we had news we would be rescued the next morning and that our son Peter in Townsville had been informed we were alive and well. We travelled on without further incident, the car and trailer caked in dried mud. We had a wonderful time with our family and returned home on the bitumen via Alice Springs.

During this travel adventure, I started feeling different somehow. I spoke to Allan about the pressing need I had been feeling to give something back, and also told him about the strange vision of me holding a black baby that had kept reappearing day after day until I just accepted it. Allan listened as I explained and then suggested I talk to one of our ministers when we got home.

It is difficult to describe the next events in my spiritual journey, but I did feel the need to start writing down what was happening to me and all the thoughts and feelings I was wrestling with. One night I awoke at two in the morning with these words loud and forceful in my head: My soul magnifies the Lord. I eventually went back to sleep wondering what was happening. The next night at 3 am I was again woken, this time with the words: I will lift up my eyes unto the hills – where does my help come from?

I now know these verses are from Luke 1:47 and Psalm 121. They have since become very important and symbolic to me but, at the time, not being a reader of the Bible, I didn't know what they meant or where they came from. As a child at the convent we had sung the Magnificat: 'My soul glorifies the Lord' but that was a very long time ago. I looked up a concordance in Allan's Bible to find out what Jesus was saying to me. The more I read, the more the Psalms started speaking to me. I stopped watching television and read the Bible, books on spirituality, autobiographies – anything that taught me more.

Before this time I had never concentrated seriously on prayer but it was around then that I had two powerful experiences with it. In both instances my prayers concerned problems affecting friends, one who required physical healing and the other vital help in beating her children's serious drug addiction. In both cases my prayers were answered dramatically and almost instantly, which left me breathless. Then there was a more personal answer to prayer.

During a routine ophthalmic check-up, a specialist diagnosed a rapidly growing cataract in my left eye. I presumed that if God wanted me working overseas then he would deal with it, and so I prayed to that effect. I sought a second opinion and, after an examination, the specialist said, 'There is nothing wrong with your eye.' Discussing this later with a medical colleague, he declared there was no way the first diagnosis could have been a mistake.

I began to feel that I was needed somewhere in the world and had a very strong feeling it was in India or Africa. I felt I had been called and it didn't feel negotiable. Asking 'why?' or 'what for?' didn't occur to me, but I did want to ask 'why me?'

I was aware of my other responsibilities as a wife, mother and grandmother, but Allan took each step with me. He liked the change he saw in me and encouraged me to follow the call.

I took Allan's advice and met one of the ministers at Westbourne Park Uniting Church, which we had been attending since Allan retired. It was a busy place with several hundred people at the two morning services. One day I sat down in the church office with Reverend Gillies Ambler and told him that I felt a calling to work with children and babies in India or Africa, and that I wanted him to help me discover where. Gillies was slightly taken aback by my directness, but importantly he was immediately open to the idea. Although he knew little about working in such places, he offered to help find out.

In the meantime, Gillies began nudging this spiritual awakening I was experiencing in all sorts of directions. He urged me to explore and reflect on where it was leading me and arranged mini-retreats to read and reflect. Gillies is a bit of a maverick in spiritual matters and believes God doesn't always follow orthodox or well-trodden paths. He was open to anywhere this might lead, but also warned that this would mean letting go of control of many things – something that doesn't come naturally to me.

Despite having said I did not want to be a volunteer, Allan and I started going out with the Salvation Army each week on their soup run. I felt needed and was helping people in distress. We drove up and down streets in the city looking for the homeless and hungry and giving them something to eat and warm clothes. It was humbling learning from those who had nothing. One old man had been a Second World War Russian pilot; we affectionately called him The General. I was told that once his parachute had not opened properly and he had suffered multiple fractures, so consequently his life was filled with pain. I don't know what happened to him – he just disappeared.

Three months after my outback vision, I was feeling restless at work. I believed that at fifty-five I had achieved all I wanted to at Resthaven and something was calling me away. I surprised everyone at work when I announced my retirement, but I couldn't really answer their questions about what I was going to do – I really didn't know, but I wanted to start whatever it was immediately.

We began looking for mission agencies, but doors seemed to be closing rather than opening. Some suggested training, others language school. Some didn't know of anywhere in Africa and referred me to the Philippines, but that didn't feel right. I sensed strongly that my calling would involve children and presumed that meant working in an orphanage. Wherever it was, I felt convinced it would involve only one overseas visit and then I would resume my retired life.

After about six months I heard of a couple from the Adelaide Hills, Frank and Michele Heyward, who were going to Uganda in east Africa to build a school, church and clinic. They were completely self-funded: Frank would do the building while

Michele would handle the administration and keep the books. I contacted them a few weeks before they left and discussed their plans. They invited me to live with them if I came to Uganda. While there was nothing I could do for the Heywards, Michele told me about a place called the Florence Nightingale Clinic in Nakalubye which she described as the worst slum in Kampala. It was run by a nurse who she said would be grateful for any assistance. The only thing I knew about Uganda was the terrifying years under the rule of Idi Amin but now it seemed politically stable. This seemed the clearest lead I had to work overseas. I still had no real plan, place to work or obvious use of my skills, but it was a start.

For the next six months I did Bible study at Tabor College, a theological college in Adelaide. Although I didn't complete the course, I felt it was important to learn about the Bible and how to read meaning into the lessons it taught. I also undertook an intensive course in international health and medicine run by Flinders University Emeritus Professor Anthony Radford, a beautiful man who became a friend and mentor. His overseas experience was extraordinary having worked in forty-six countries, including stints in Papua New Guinea, Alaska, Botswana, China, Burma and refugee camps on the Thai–Cambodia border. Along the way he has met Mother Theresa, Prince Charles and Jawaharlal Nehru.

Anthony's intense three-week course, the only one of its type in Australia, is designed to prepare Christian medical professionals for work in developing countries. Anthony is a great believer in holistic medicine and argues that the best way to tackle illness in developing countries is not with a single doctor, but with a plan to educate and alleviate poverty. Simple things such as hand-washing, birth control, teeth-cleaning and mosquito nets will change many more people's lives than a team of specialist surgeons. Often these basic health principles are not carried out because of ignorance, illiteracy or poverty. The course emphasised the role community health workers can play, because Anthony's experience is that the only sustainable programs are ones that can be taught to others, not just implemented by a foreigner who jets into a community.

Between Anthony's crash courses in leprosy, malaria, basic dentistry, nutrition, STDs and dysentery were lessons in self-preservation. There is a very high burn-out rate for Westerners going into developing countries. Anthony warned stress levels could quickly reach the point where I would forget how to phone home and advised taking a book of phone numbers and instructions on how to dial international codes. He taught us some ways to alleviate the intense homesickness, such as keeping a journal.

Our final project was to break into groups and come up with a community health project, setting an objective and developing a plan of action. Anthony emphasised plans that galvanise a community into action and setting goals that can be measured. Although the course was jammed into three demanding weeks, so many of the aspects, good and bad, that were discussed in theory in it would become reality in Uganda.

The next few months sped by quickly. I had thought about what to take with me to give to the children of Nakulabye so I decided to collect t-shirts. With the help of friends from church we gathered about 200 brightly coloured t-shirts. Michele asked the nurse at the Florence Nightingale clinic what instruments or drugs I could bring. I collected what I could from Overseas Pharmaceutical Aid for Life (OPAL), a South Australian charity started by a former police officer Geoff Lockyer, who was outraged at the amount of surplus but safe medicines in Australia dumped by companies. He began collecting the excess and has provided drugs for clinics and hospitals in more than forty countries.

I had retired in October 1998 and by the following April I was at the Adelaide airport nervously saying goodbye to Allan. I had to fly to Perth from where I would fly to Harare in Zimbabwe and then, after two days, onto Uganda. I still knew very little about this country, what to expect from its people or how I could help, if at all.

Chapter Three

ON THE FLIGHT FROM Perth to Zimbabwe I was given a rare treat by being allowed up to the flight deck. The first officer knew my son David from RAAF days and they were both now flying for Qantas. It was terrific to be able to see where he sits and works. When I returned to my seat I found myself getting emotional as I read through a very moving letter that our church minister, Gillies, had written to me, and I hit an internal panic button about what lay ahead. I opened my Bible for comfort and told myself to trust and obey.

I had a stopover in Harare because Uganda Airways only had one plane and the next scheduled flight to Uganda was in two days. Peter Burkett from the International Police Association (IPA) met me at Harare airport and helped collect my things. Allan is also a member of the IPA, a worldwide organisation whose members offer support and assistance to police officers and their families when travelling. I had checked in with me a box of medication from OPAL. Irritatingly, the package was nowhere to be seen. We spent ages trying to locate it until someone finally told us it was now coming from Singapore via Johannesburg. I was having my first rapid course in how things do (or don't) work in Africa.

The morning I flew to Uganda I was a bundle of nerves. Regular visits to the loo began at 4 am, and eventually I took some medication, made myself eat some peaches and drink some black tea, and calm myself down by praying. Although still a bit fearful, about halfway through the flight I was overcome by an incredible sense of peace, no doubt a combination of the prayer and the medication!

Entebbe airport near Kampala, the Ugandan capital on Lake Victoria, was all but empty as I walked through customs. I told one of the officers that I wasn't sure if I had to declare anything and he replied, 'No, madame, you do not, and I will push your trolley for you.' He held the door open as I sailed through with my case, two boxes, t-shirts for the children, a carry-on bag and a laundry bag full of books.

'Hallelujah,' I whispered to myself.

Outside the terminal I was met by a welcoming party led by Frank and Michele Heyward and their teenage daughter, Hannah. The Heywards have three children but two were grown up and stayed in Australia. Although I had only met them briefly in Australia and didn't become involved with their work, they opened their home to me to stay and we became great friends. I was introduced to a woman named Alice Zalawango who was about forty, and very excited to meet me. She ran the Florence

Nightingale Clinic and was, for better or worse, to become my clinic nurse and teacher of all things Ugandan for the next three months.

The twenty-kilometre drive from Entebbe to the Heywards' house took over an hour as we battled the traffic along poor roads. As we bumped over the pot holes, I naively asked where the footpaths were. There are no footpaths anywhere in Uganda apart from the inner city. There was rubbish piled high and plastic bags everywhere. I was shocked to see so many coffins waiting to be sold. There are more than one million people in Kampala and it felt like all of them were on the road. Drivers used their horns liberally, and road rules seemed to be used merely as suggestions with cars, motorbikes and *boda-bodas* darting in and out at all angles and speeds. *Boda-bodas* are small motorbikes, similar to scooters, and are the most popular (and hair-raising) way of getting around. Frank said the roads were in quite good condition. My overwhelming impression of the city was stark poverty.

The Heywards' house was in a rural area north of Kampala. My plan was to live there for three months. Michele had gone to a lot of trouble to make my room pretty with curtains and matching bedspread. The house was very simple with cement floors and primitive facilities, but it was safe. I had already heard stories about Uganda's crime rate and the perils of being alone, particularly at night. The indoor flush toilet was accessed through their bedroom, so a pit latrine in the backyard was the alternative. Next door an orphanage owned by an American housed twenty-two gorgeous children being cared for by five 'aunties', each child being funded by an American sponsor. The children regularly made their way into the Heywards' house along with other boisterous visitors, so I had to quickly get used to the lack of privacy.

Once a woman named Edith arrived to see Michele, and when I introduced myself her response was to ask me if I was saved. She was the first of many Ugandans I would meet whose faith was a powerful force. Christianity is the dominant religion in Uganda but there are also Muslims and those with traditional indigenous beliefs. I quickly learned whatever the religion, this is a deeply spiritual country. It was explained to me that so many lost so much under the brutal regimes of Presidents Idi Amin and Milton Obote that they were sustained by their faith which they clung to fiercely. Over time I discovered how freely Ugandans talk about God and the spirit. This wasn't restricted to Christians as Muslims were equally passionate about the power of God in their lives.

My first experience with Christianity Ugandan-style, at a church in a Kampala suburb with about 2000 in the congregation, was an eye-opener. I went along with the Heywards, who worshipped here until their own church was built. The service lasted three hours; I was later told this was a short service so I made a mental note to bring something to eat and drink next time. The music and singing was beautiful and reflected the love of the congregation so much that I found myself immersed in the spirituality of the moment. However the atmosphere changed for me when the sermon began and a woman screeched from the pulpit for almost an hour. I'm familiar with evangelism, but this would take some getting used to. Eventually I moved away from the Pentecostal-style services, preferring instead the Church of Uganda which was Anglican and its services were in English. In a week the church was to be used for the wedding of a friend of the Heywards', Fred, and his fiancée, Florence, with the reception to be held in the garden at Frank and Michele's home. The couple already had three children and their fourth was due in three months. It is so expensive for Ugandans to get married that many can't afford it. I was automatically invited to the wedding because I was a friend of the Heywards so, as per the local custom, I gave the couple 20,000 shillings (A$20) which sent Fred into a speech of praise to God.

Before anyone can marry in Uganda, they must have what is called the 'introduction'. It is more important than the wedding itself because it involves paying a dowry. This wedding introduction began with a bone-crushing drive to Florence's village, where there had been much work done erecting a shelter and bringing chairs in for us. The men were formally dressed in long, white robes called *kunzu* and suit coats, while the women looked elegant in their traditional dresses known as a *gomez*. It has many metres of fabric which are folded over and over in a pleat on the left side and held in place by a bright brocade sash. I decided I needed to get a *gomez* and some dangling earrings from the market for such occasions.

The introduction ceremony took hours and there was much drama, play-acting and Bible reading. Florence came in looking splendid, surrounded by her sisters and aunt. She did not speak to Fred and he was not allowed to say anything all day. Eventually we were served a meal of meat soup, beans, greens and rice, served on a banana leaf and eaten by hand. A girl came around both before and after the meal with water to wash our hands.

The wedding was held in a church in Kampala the following day, so we decorated Frank's car with bandages made from old sheets and tied bougainvillea to it. I was getting used to the flexible nature of African time and the phrase 'TIA' – 'This is Africa' – often uttered when things run behind schedule. The wedding was supposed to be at one o'clock but it was 1.45 when twelve of us piled into the Pajero and took Fred to the church. We need not have hurried because Florence arrived at 3.30 and the ceremony went until five. The reception at Frank and Michele's was a riot of colour and music, with three different singing groups and many speeches. It ended with ten guests sleeping on the lounge room floor.

A few days later I went with Michele to meet Alice at the Florence Nightingale Clinic to see if I could help in any way. My feelings were mixed. I was excited, nervous and wondering what I was doing here. The 24-hour clinic stands in the middle of the Nakulabye slum. It is a seething mass of humanity where 80,000 people live in poverty and sickness. When it rains it turns into a bog, the open sewerage drains overflow and rubbish that is never collected piles up.

The clinic's work mostly revolved around mothers and babies but occasionally people with minor wounds would be attended to or those who suspected they had AIDS or STDs would come in to talk discreetly to Alice about it. The clinic delivery room was about two metres by one, with a cement floor, screened area and a battered examination couch. In another passageway was a mattress where the mother could rest for eight to twelve hours after delivery. I was told most births take place at home and only the problems end up at the clinic, but in reality there were many normal deliveries there. The bathroom was a pit latrine out the back. Alice had spread the word about my arrival and many mothers came to see me, asking for advice for their children and themselves. They pushed their babies forward for treatment and I immunised some as young as five days old with vaccines that were readily available. I found myself terrified at the responsibility.

One worried woman arrived with her ten-month-old son, William, who had lost a lot of weight. His chest was rattly and he had a rapid pulse. I knew he had a chest infection and needed antibiotics, but they were back at the house, the only medications I had were cough mixture and Panadol. I should have picked him up and taken him with his mama to a hospital but it was my first day and I didn't understand the Ugandan health system. I held the little boy and came close to tears. I asked his mother to return the next day when I would bring the medications from OPAL and she began crying. Through Alice's translation she told me she had never known caring before and thanked me for showing love to her and her baby. I realised in that helpless moment that William and others like him were the reason I was in Africa.

The next day I returned with the medications. Already the patients had started calling me *mzungu* Judy, meaning white person Judy. I held a two-week-old baby girl who was a tiny two kilos at birth, but her weight had dropped dramatically and her temperature was 40°C. I feared she was dying of pneumonia and told her mother to take her straight to hospital. The mama walked away crying while carrying her precious little scrap of humanity.

William looked a little better and his mother was smiling in her gentle way. After his first dose, she continued bringing her son to the clinic four times a day for his antibiotic mixtures. They lived in terrible conditions and although there was some improvement, William wasn't overcoming his illness. One orphaned baby was brought in by his grandmother. She could only afford to give him 'dry tea' (tea without milk) and porridge. I feared he had little hope of survival. I had to remind myself of the lesson I had been taught at Tabor College – that I can't save everybody.

A week later I was told William had died and had been buried the day before. I was sort of prepared, but I still wept for him and his mama. William was the first Ugandan baby I had held and so I desperately wanted him to live. I had come to Uganda to make a difference to a child and he had died and it was shattering. I visited his mother, Tewopisita Nalwadda or Tewo, a beautiful woman in her late twenties. To find her I walked for five minutes from the clinic through the slum. Part of the journey involved squeezing between two walls about half a metre apart while straddling an open drain; I could only imagine what it would be like when hit by tropical rain. This was my first walk deep into the slums and it was shocking. Rubbish was piled high with plastic bags full of everything, including faeces. I jumped over used condoms. The gutters were full of stagnant water and the combined smell assaulted my senses. There were tiny food stalls crammed between noisy video shops where movies were played blaring out into the street. Meat lay uncovered on wooden counters crawling with flies. Gorgeous but grubby little children ran out and touched me and ran away because I was a *mzungu* and they hadn't seen one before.

Tewo lived in a room about two metres square, with a small two-seater lounge at one end and a mat and a few pots on the concrete floor. Tewo's husband had been murdered when she was pregnant with William, and her parents and siblings were all dead. There was no-one left to comfort her and I couldn't imagine the grief and sorrow she was suffering. I felt overwhelmed by the widespread loss of human life in this country. In addition to her grief, Tewo faced eviction from her tiny room if she didn't pay the equivalent of $80 for four months rent.

Tewo visited the clinic a few hours later complaining of a headache and fever, and I suspected she was coming down with malaria.

Chapter Four

I NEEDED TO UNDERSTAND how best to treat malaria so approached Dr Edward Ssembatya who was involved with the clinic in a voluntary capacity. He had previously come to teach me about Ugandan drug laws, during which he offered to help with some of the red tape so future medications could be brought in formally and possibly in larger quantities. He was in his forties, quietly spoken and gentle, and what impressed me from the very first was his love for his fellow Ugandans and the complete respect that he showed them.

Dr Edward, as he was known, ran the Busabala Road Hospital about ten kilometres away in the suburb of Najjanankumbi, with an outpatient department and a training centre for nurses. It was a 24-hour facility open to anyone, and Dr Edward performed minor surgery and normal deliveries, but more complicated cases were transferred to a major hospital. After examining Tewo, he asked if I would visit his hospital because he wanted advice on administration. In reality he wanted advice on managing nursing staff – something which was second nature for me. I quickly discovered there were many differences between nursing staff in Uganda and Australia. Here they were paid a pittance and didn't always have a strong work ethic.

Gaining access to even the most basic medical attention is beyond the reach of most poor Ugandans, so most have to suffer in silence. While they might hope they would get better, there was a resignation about death because it was everywhere. In Australia, one in 200 babies does not see its first birthday; in Uganda, one in every ten babies die in their first year of life. The diseases that kill them are pneumonia, gastroenteritis, malaria, HIV, measles and malnutrition. But the underlying reasons for their deaths are poverty, powerlessness, and a lack of education and access to resources.

Amid this atmosphere, the idea that someone would offer even the slightest help was greeted with rejoicing. I was getting adept at catching buses and getting around Kampala. I was also learning how to bargain at the street markets and try local foods. I was missing Australian food, especially cheese, which was prohibitively expensive. I worked a full eight hours at the clinic each day, stopping for lunch of meat or fish cooked like a stew with rice or *matoke*. The Florence Nightingale Clinic staff gave me the name *Kisakye* (pronounced *chis-ar-chee*), which means grace, full of God. When they first translated it, I felt humbled: the Ugandans were offering up so much love and were so grateful for what little I could do for them. One woman in her forties came in with gynaecological problems. A doctor had told her that if she had a baby it would fix things, but I feared she had endometriosis. She already had seven children and when I asked if she wanted more, she cried, 'Definitely not.' I arranged for her to see another doctor for advice and treatment, remembering Anthony explaining that if a woman can delay becoming pregnant by a year after a birth, then it dramatically increases the chances of her next child being healthy.

Family planning seemed to be an important health issue. Patients regularly came in suffering from sexually transmitted diseases, particularly young people with syphilis. I was learning fast about the sexual habits of Ugandans. Girls aged as young as ten will prostitute themselves for the equivalent of ten cents. When I asked one of the young Muslim nurses at the clinic about how young people deal with and understand HIV she replied, 'During the day we remember but at night we forget.' Husbands go away looking for work and have unprotected sex and then come home and infect their wives. Rape is a common crime. There was a desperate need for an STD clinic, not only for treatment but to explain the diseases and how they could be prevented from spreading.

One day, after a busy morning, it started raining so by mid afternoon the clinic was empty. I went with Alice to visit Tewo. She greeted me by calling me her mother, and I called her my other daughter. I had been thinking about how I could help her, so I gave her money for food and an offer of A$20 to establish a business selling second-hand clothes in the market. I wanted to keep the offer quiet so I wouldn't be inundated with others looking for money, but I also made it clear I wanted a weekly update on how things were going.

The next day I went with Alice and a clinic nurse named Recheal to see Tewo's landlord, as he had come to Tewo's house and announced he wanted her to move to another room because hers needed renovating. I insisted on inspecting the new room and found it was filthy, with no window, lock or door handle, and backing onto a video room where the locals watched movies. As the TV blared out full-blast at 10.30 in the morning, I told him I was not allowing her to be shifted into this room. The landlord followed us back to Tewo's and sat down on the couch, and for some reason I asked Alice to enquire if he believed in Jesus. He replied he did and that he was born again, so I asked him to treat Tewo with respect and a gentleness as Jesus would have. To my amazement this turned things around, and he wrote in her rent book that he and his family would accept greater responsibility for her to live safely and, when the time came to renovate her room, they would ensure she had appropriate and free alternative accommodation until it was ready. I promised him I would pay the next four months rent when the renovation was complete, being able to give Tewo this start with a donation that friends in Australia had given me before I left.

My visits to the clinic usually began with a series of hair-raising taxi rides. Taxis in Kampala operate like a minibus service and take as many passengers as they can squeeze in. It was best just to shut my eyes and pray when the driver hit the accelerator and launched into the traffic. I have no idea how they manoeuvre their vehicles into the spaces they do.

I had slipped into the role of Alice's assistant very easily. I meant a lot of kudos for her because a *mzungu* was rarely seen in Nakulabye. My time was spent visiting those with AIDS and generally helping in the clinic.

Once a week Edward came to consult, and fortunately he was on hand one morning when an eighteen-month-old was brought in who was fitting and had a temperature of thirty-nine. Edward diagnosed malaria; if he hadn't been there, the child would have died. A week later the mother returned with the baby, who appeared fully recovered and sat on my knee, bouncing and laughing.

Another baby was brought into the clinic when he was about two months old and dying of pneumonia. Little Fred was filthy and had only one set of clothes, and he desperately needed help. I gave his mama the money to get him to hospital and, after he came home, she brought him to the clinic every day for me to check. It was a joy to see him thrive and grow into a gorgeous little boy.

Edward's presence made such an enormous difference that it confirmed my growing concern that this clinic didn't follow basic primary health care principles. There was a pattern of dangerous practices such as multiple babies being immunised with the same needles. In addition to delivering and immunising babies there was some counselling for those with HIV/AIDS, but mostly they just referred people on and gave out paracetamol. Although I was not running the clinic I felt responsible for the correct handling of the drugs I had brought from Australia. I discovered one of the nurse aide's had dispensed medications which I had specifically said were not to be – there was no harm done but the lack of understanding frustrated me. I arranged for a cupboard to be built so medications could be locked away.

In addition to the operational aspects, I was confused by the structure, financing and accountability of the clinic. I couldn't get straight answers on these matters, other than that the clinic existed on donations and minimal payments from some patients (the equivalent of ten to fifty cents per visit) and that the staff were volunteers. The electricity was regularly cut off and I couldn't find out if it was because of non-payment or dodgy wiring. One day, two packets of examination gloves appeared which were labelled as free from UNESCO; this bonus was treated as an example of how the clinic operated on donations. When I asked Alice who gave what from where and how or if things were paid for, her answers were elusive. I was to discover this was normal with her and eventually I came to believe I was being lied to. This frustrated me greatly because the lack of accountability seemed to be reflected in the nursing. I decided I wouldn't make any more commitments until I got to the bottom line. I would not be used.

I decided to take up Edward's invitation to visit his hospital in Najjanankumbi. He sent his car to collect us and I went with Alice and two of her nurses. At first I was appalled at the tiny eight bed hospital. Edward greeted us in his modest, sparsely furnished office. The nurses from the Nakulabye clinic were brought there for experience and worked eight- to ten-hour days, seven days per week. They were paid very little, if at all, but had accommodation and food.

Patients at the hospital paid a fee for treatment and medication. Through these funds Edward had built the tiny hospital, but he had bigger plans and construction was under way on a new thirty-bed hospital next door. The work was going ahead in fits and starts, depending on Edward's income; when he could afford to buy some bricks, the next section would begin construction. The plans were eventually for a three-storey building designed around a central open courtyard. It was still just a shell with a roof, and lacked plumbing, electricity, doors and flyscreens.

I had no idea what lay ahead for this hospital, nor how it would change so many lives over the next few years both in Uganda and Australia.

Chapter Five

ALTHOUGH MOST OF THE work at the Florence Nightingale Clinic was with mothers and babies, I was soon confronted by my first AIDS case. Timothy, a man aged about thirty in an advanced stage of the illness came in, anxious and desperate. I could do nothing for him medically – the expensive drugs available to HIV patients in the West were unavailable to the poor in Africa – but we talked about his condition and his life. The longer we spoke, the more he relaxed. I promised I would visit Timothy at home after work at the clinic. After he left I was surprised at how close to God I felt and that I had been given the right words to say. I continued to visit Timothy regularly and we became friends. He died a few weeks later and I realised with sadness that this was going to be the norm. I would just get to know someone and then they would die. I was grateful for my faith because it helped me cope. I found much-needed peace in the Bible, reminding myself that God loved the poor, sick and the lame and I knew he also loved these poor beautiful people who were dying of AIDS.

HIV/AIDS is the plague of Africa. It does not discriminate between rich and poor, old or young, and the stigma attached to it has frustrated public health efforts. While the epidemic spread across the Western world, by the late 1980s public health education and pharmaceuticals began slowing its progress. But in sub-Saharan Africa, the most heavily affected region in the world, there were an estimated 22 million HIV cases by 2007, with that number growing by almost 2 million per year. It is almost impossible to describe the toll the infection takes on communities. The additional heartbreak is to see innocents infected: more than 90 per cent of new HIV infections among children are transferred from mother to child. Half of those children born HIV-positive will die before their second birthday. In some remote areas of Uganda, unofficially up to 90 per cent of the adult population is HIV-positive. There are lost generations, with the very old looking after the very young. All those in-between have died of AIDS.

While some Africa governments have ignored AIDS, Uganda has curbed the spread, but this is not to suggest it hasn't taken an enormous toll on the nation. The first case was diagnosed in 1982 and by the mid 1990s, 15 per cent of adults were HIV-positive. In 1986 the Ugandan Government made its first effort to control the spread of the disease, and President Museveni went on a national tour promoting what was called the 'ABC campaign', which had as its message:

Abstain from sex before marriage
Be faithful to your partner and use
Condoms.

By the late 1990s the number of cases seemed to be on the way down, but the terrible time lag between infection and death meant that, even if halted overnight, the damage already caused would be felt for decades to come.

Those with AIDS in Uganda suffer terribly as their condition deteriorates. I visited one man named Katumba who had moved out of his house because his wife was having difficulty taking care of him. His pain was out of control, he was restless and she was frightened. He was living with his son and sleeping on a ragged mattress on the floor. No-one was really caring for him (although his wife did visit) and his bedding was full of grit corroding from the adjacent sandstone wall. He had been visited by nurses from Mengo Hospital, one of the major hospitals in Kampala, who had left some pretty useless pills. I gave him some more effective medication, cleaned him up and tried to make him comfortable and prayed with him. Katumba died the next day.

One day a young man called Dennis, who was the youth representative on the Nakulabye Council, asked me to visit his best friend. Jeffrey was twenty-eight years old and in the final stages of AIDS. He lived with his wife, Jennifer, and their ten-year-old son. Having worked in a hospice in Adelaide for several years, I thought I had seen every awful kind of death – but I was wrong. Jeffrey was dying in abject poverty and I had never seen such horrible bedsores; Jeffrey's sacral area at the base of his spine was rotting flesh, right down to the bone – the wound was the size of a dinner plate. I asked Edward for some pethidine for the pain and bought a large bag of rice for Jennifer so they had something to eat. I visited twice a day and sometimes nurses from the clinic would come. We sponged him and at times he seemed almost unconscious and peaceful while this was going on. Then he would break out violently, shouting and screaming. Once he yelled, 'Break the chains that bind me,' and so we prayed and everyone in the room joined in. All I had left was prayer. I was so frustrated and angry that I could not do more for this suffering man. In the end I just cried. I had no more narcotics and so bought intramuscular valium from a chemist and gave it to him, promising to return in two hours. When I did he had rested and taken some nourishment. He opened his eyes and said *kale* – thank you.

As I left Dennis was waiting, but this time he asked me to visit his mother who he said was very sick. When I arrived at her house it was so small and dark that I could barely see her lying in bed. Someone lit a tiny paraffin flame and told me she had suffered from malaria plus a loss of weight and severe coughing. I suspected a combination of tuberculosis and AIDS, so I gave her chloroquine tablets for the malaria.

As I left and weaved my way back through the tiny alleyways between the slums, little children shouted out to me and some men called out *kisakye webale webale nnyo*. Recheal translated it as 'miracle grace from God, thank you very much for what you are doing'. Over the next few days, Edward gave me more pethidine to give Jeffrey some relief. When he died, three days later, I felt grateful his suffering had ended and that he had at least had two or three peaceful days in his final week.

After only a month in Uganda I realised I needed some time on my own. The days in the clinic were exhausting; not only the rush of people wanting help but also adjusting to the heat, language and cultural subtleties of Uganda. I missed Allan desperately and craved letters from home, as well as simple things like bread. In Uganda, bread is sweet and made with loads of sugar, though eventually I found a bakery that made bread with salt.

I was very tired at night, and coming home to a house constantly full of visitors and neighbouring orphans wasn't helping me rest. One morning I answered a knock on the door at home to find a nurse from the clinic who had tracked me down and wanted 800,000 shillings (A$700) for sponsorship. Being asked for this type of assistance was to become a regular occurrence, but I learned quickly how to say no. Another time there was a robbery next door and we were awoken by screaming. Unfortunately it wasn't unusual to hear screams in Kampala at night due to domestic violence, but in this case there had been six armed intruders and a man was stabbed.

The heavy tropical rains made things even more difficult. One morning after it rained, I made my way to the clinic through ankle-deep mud, remaining upright until the last minute. As I fell, my shoe stuck in the mud and my foot flew out and landed in a bog. The incident seemed to aggravate something in my knee and it would often bother me at night, despite applying heat rub. Edward arranged an X-ray of my knee which cleared it of any breaks but I began taking anti-inflammatory medication to ease the pain. I missed my life in Adelaide and was struggling to come to terms with the reason for my being in Uganda. What difference could I, a fifty-six-year-old retired nurse, possibly make? I was homesick for my man, my house, my family and friends and everything I had taken for granted for so long. I wondered if I was making a difference at all. In hindsight I realised this breaking point was the beginning of what was my apprenticeship in Uganda.

In an attempt to counter these feelings, I booked into the Sheraton Hotel for a night. I had no problem dealing with the luxury because one of the things I had learned at my brief training was the importance of going somewhere like this to take time out. Despite being right in the centre of the city, the hotel is surrounded by beautiful gardens and my room had a wonderful view, soft pillows, carpet and lights that stayed on (when you wanted them to). In addition to the hospitality there was the added attraction of a functioning business centre, so I immediately sent and received emails. Allan rang twice and it was wonderful to hear his voice and talk to him. Later I had calls from Peter, Fiona and David.

I wallowed in twenty-four hours of luxury, beginning with a haircut and head massage. Then I climbed into a huge hot bath and read my book while sipping on a glass of wine. The television in my room wasn't working but I didn't care, instead watching a stunning sunset and looking at my photo album which I had brought from home. In the evening I ate in the restaurant but found I couldn't finish my steak; I suspect I was now unused to eating so much. At lunch on Sunday I discovered several other expatriates enjoying the buffet after church – it seems the Sheraton is a regular place for mini-retreats.

My return to the reality of Uganda came two days later when I visited a village church. Frank and Michele were involved there and were assisting the local pastor. They invited me to visit to see if I could instigate some treatment for the children who were all suffering from malnutrition, worms and chest infections. It was on the outer edge of Nakulabye, not far from a trading centre and marketplace along a potholed dirt road. The bins trailing one side of the road were overflowing with decaying rubbish, children searching through them for something to eat. The Wall of Fire Church was built out of rusty sheets of corrugated iron, plastic bags and papyrus reeds. Four people were living in the back of the church in desperate conditions: an 87-year-old woman and her 60-year-old daughter in one room and in another partitioned area was a small nine-year-old girl named Beth and her mother, Anna-Mary. The two older women suffered whenever it rained because both the roof and the walls leaked, so water ran through their room.

Before I left Adelaide I had been given some money by an Adelaide Rotary Club with the freedom to use it where I thought the need greatest. In my heart I couldn't think of a more worthy recipient so I arranged for their room to be rebuilt, evicting six rats along the way. We had enough money left over to buy a single bed and mattress which the two women shared, and they were so excited they both hugged me. We also began working on a plan to help Beth get to school.

Beth had been to stay with Frank and Michele for a few days and when I got up one morning she had washed all the floors. I felt this little girl needed a chance to go to school. The Heywards were starting a sponsorship program supported by their church in Australia. In the years to come the organisation would set up formal sponsorship for hundreds of orphans, leading them to build their own church and school. I sent home an email to Allan suggesting we sponsor Beth and he agreed so we began by arranging for her to visit a dentist, which turned out to be something of a disaster as she screamed the house down and wouldn't let the dentist near her. He was at least able to catch sight of her teeth, which needed fillings and three extractions. Afterwards the dentist began discussing fees until I explained her living conditions and that I had taken on the responsibility of her support, and he (bless him) said he would waive all fees. Her mother, Anna-Mary, brought her back the following week and Beth behaved and her teeth were fixed.

A few weeks later we drove over the most tortuous non-existent roads to enrol Beth and a boy named Gerard (who was being sponsored by Frank and Michele) at school. They were so excited about starting the next day. I bought them a couple of extra reading and writing books and the teacher offered to give them extra tuition for a fee. It was so wonderful to see Beth's face glued to the window of her classroom with a look of excitement and anticipation. My mind raced, thinking about what potential lay ahead for this nine-year-old. Would we be supporting her right through to university?

Over the next few weeks in the clinic, news of my work spread through Nakulabye. A cheeky little three-year-old named Thomas and his band of merry friends popped in and out crying, 'Mama Jude loves me.' Thomas lived next door to the clinic with his mother, who had a small street stall selling vegetables and dried fish, while his father had died from AIDS. Thomas decided that he loved me, and I certainly loved him. Thomas would sit on a stool and watch me work for hours on end, even as babies screamed during immunisations. Little children like him captured my heart, and it did my soul good to cuddle a healthy baby. After one visit to Jeffrey, I came into the clinic to see Thomas standing on the steps, declaring in a bossy voice, 'Mama Jude is back and she loves me.' His sidekick, Karlim, slipped in quietly to see me on his own. This day he was wearing a shirt and, I noticed with a smile, trousers that actually stayed up.

Chapter Six

DESPITE HAVING MUCH TO occupy myself with, I was still unsure what my future work in Africa would involve, if anything. I wasn't prepared to commit myself to the clinic because I felt unclear about its role beyond immunisations and midwifery, worthwhile as these were. I worried both that the nurses were not being trained properly and about the accounting. The staff were not using aseptic techniques, the basic method of preventing contamination by using sterile equipment and fluids during nursing procedures. As far as I could tell, they could all have become HIV-positive because of a lack of basic medical education. It was a big decision to commit myself financially, physically and emotionally to something that I had so many questions about. The worries left me fearful, tired and feeling a little sorry for myself.

Eventually there was no choice but to speak candidly to Edward and Alice about my concerns. I had been in the city and we had arranged a meeting at the clinic. After catching three mini-buses and walking almost two kilometres to the meeting place, Alice told me things were busy and the meeting was off. I was feeling frustrated on my walk back to the taxi until I had a delightful encounter with an old lady. She was walking with difficulty, but still the conductor wouldn't let her get onto the taxi because she was the equivalent of twenty cents short of the fare. I paid the fare and told him quite firmly to put her off at the right place. When we sat down together on the bus I nearly suffocated (the poor woman was extremely odorous) but we shared the biscuits I had in my bag and chatted, with others on the bus interpreting. By the time I got off everyone knew what I was doing, where I was from and the answer to the insistent question: where is your husband?

After being in Uganda for a month, my administrative skills were starting to be recognised. I was approached to meet medical officers and nurse educators at Kampala's Mengo Hospital, established by the British medical missionaries Sir Albert and Katherine Cook in 1897 and the oldest in East Africa. Sir Albert's vision was to create a maternity training school in Kampala and so he wrote training manuals in the Ugandan language, Luganda. Although English, and to a lesser degree Swahili, is widely used in Uganda, Luganda is the language of the slums and among the illiterate. Katherine was matron of both the hospital and, later, a nurses' training college. Sir Albert later started the Mulago Hospital, to treat venereal diseases and sleeping disorders, and another school for training Ugandan medical officers. Katherine died in 1938 while Sir Albert passed away in Kampala in 1951. The Mengo Hospital continues to be run with the help of a small British charity, while the Mulago has grown into the largest teaching hospital in the region. It is now government owned and operated and includes institutes for heart, cancer, infectious diseases, burns and plastic surgery.

There is no access to Mengo if you don't pay. While there has always been access for the poor to Mulago Hospital, this works in a vastly different way to anything I had ever known. Patients must take their own carer, bedding, bowls and food, and pay for medication. On my visit I was impressed with how Mengo was run and we effectively had a brain-storming session. I suggested the need for a course for village nurse aides who were trained in primary health care. We spoke about concentrating the care in the village and preventing illness from occurring rather than having to treat it.

The next day I met Lawrence Kaggwa, medical director of the Mulago Hospital. When I arrived at his office he had only five minutes scheduled. After I hastily told him my qualifications and experience, his manner changed and he offered many apologies and insisted we meet again in a week. As he left he arranged for a nurse to give me a guided tour of the hospital, considered the finest in Uganda.

It was shock time for Judy! Apart from the ward sister, I didn't see a nurse in any ward. The postnatal ward was so crowded there were mums and babies sitting on the terrazzo floor; there weren't even mattresses let alone beds. I visited accident and emergency to see how things functioned when I sent a mother from the clinic. It was overcrowded with long lines of patients waiting to be seen. It was a huge challenge to my previous training and experience in casualty at the Royal Adelaide Hospital. There was very little evidence of medical supplies and chaos seemed to rule everywhere. Toward the end of my tour I cuddled a precious little boy who had been brought to the hospital after being abandoned, tossed down a pit latrine. When he was rescued he had maggots in his ears. After I got home I sat down and reflected on the day, realising that I had to come to terms quickly with the sadness of this country and that there would be some things I could never change.

A week later I met Dr Kaggwa again, but this time for an hour. He was interested in my work and asked if I would write up something on caring for him to use in teaching his staff and to show to the Ministry of Health. I promised to do so when I returned to Australia. Caring was something I had taught my nurses in Australia and I was excited to think that he would want his staff to learn this because I certainly had not seen any evidence of it. The staff were few in number and it was obvious that they were removed from anyone who was in distress. It seemed that they didn't know how to reach out and touch someone, empathy was nonexistent. I wanted to teach them the value of touching, of kindness and compassion. In reality, when I returned to Australia I wrote to Dr Kaggwa for more information before I put in the work writing up a paper, but he never replied.

The longer I was in Kampala, the more I ached for news from home. Days turned into weeks without any mail until finally I went to the post office to check if there was a reason nothing had been delivered. They took my details and promised to call, though they never did.

As I left the post office, a thief snatched my gold cross chain from around my neck in an instant. I sat down on a wall near the centre of the city and cried out of shock and fright. I wanted Allan and I wanted to go home and, briefly, I felt I had had enough of Uganda. Some passing people were very apologetic, including one lady named Sophia who stopped and talked. She was a nurse, on her way to working in a clinic that was just past mine, so we walked together. My feelings of self-pity were put into perspective as I looked around: nearby a leper sat, with damaged legs, no toes and only thumbs left on his hands. I forgave the robber and the next day five letters and a tape arrived in the post.

One day, Edward sent his driver, Abdu, and Alice to collect Michele and me. Edward had never held a driver's license and so always had a driver working for him. Apparently Edward was concerned that my view of Kampala was of an enormous slum and he was determined to show me what else the capital had to offer. We drove to the museum and then the Bugandan Parliament. Uganda has a long history of inter-tribal animosity, and the Buganda tribe (to which Edward belongs) is the largest. All the different tribes have their hierarchy, but because the Bugandan tribe is based in the Kampala area, their Parliament sits in the capital. One example of the destruction caused by the tribal warfare was the king's palace, which was in mid restoration after being bombed during the previous Obote regime.

Our last stop was the fabulous wildlife park at Entebbe, stocked with leopards, crocodiles and a majestic lion. We had a personal tour with Sam, one of the horticulturalists, who showed us how they were teaching children to save the planet Ugandan-style by growing herbal medicines. Sam told us that the monkeys here know what herbs to eat to cure themselves of malaria and worms and right on cue one performed for us, standing and beating his chest and bossing his women around.

On another day out with Edward I saw his commitment to helping others. After he and Abdu collected me in the morning, we drove 100 kilometres to a village not far from the shores of Lake Victoria. Alice and two nurses came along as well. All the local mums were waiting with their babies ready for immunisation along with some very sick people needing treatment. They had no doctor in the area although the clinic was managed by Agatha, a trained community nurse. Edward worked all day and then sat down with the mothers to educate them about HIV/AIDS, convulsions, nutrition and family planning.

I spent the day visiting people in their homes. One woman in her fifties had AIDS, as did another in her thirties who had eleven children. I was totally charmed by a seven-year-old deaf boy whose mother had Kaposi's sarcoma (cancer of the blood vessels commonly associated with AIDS). The day ended with a visit to the shores of Lake Victoria where we bought Nile perch. We got enough for everyone and took mine home to Frank and Michele's, where it was sliced into cutlets and pan fried until it was moist and succulent and then served with chips for supper.

Later that week Edward showed me more of his country, this time via a meeting with the Prime Minister of Buganda, Mulwanyamuli Semwogerere. Edward warned he would be making a donation and suggested I also make a small donation towards the forthcoming marriage of the King. I found the amount he suggested – 50,000 shillings or A$50, a small fortune to most Ugandans – hard to digest but ended up going along with it.

The Prime Minister was charming during our twenty-minute meeting. I told him of the increasing numbers of abandoned babies and the need for formula to feed them, as well as the greater numbers of people coming for advice about AIDS. The clinic was developing a reputation for treating patients kindly and with respect, and I mentioned to the Prime Minister that perhaps this was a good news story the papers could run about the clinic and the need for formula for babies. The next day I read my name in the paper for presenting the Prime Minister with 50,000 shillings towards the King's wedding. The paper also reported I came from Austria – not quite the story I had in mind.

After the meeting I went with Edward to his home village of Najjanankumbi, where he was building his hospital. The village seemed typical of what I had seen in Kampala; in five square kilometres the population is 40,000, with people living in often desperate circumstances. Edward returned to his work in the hospital. Alice had come along with one of her nurses and accompanied by two local widows we visited the aged and abandoned women of the village and those dying from AIDS.

Little did I realise that this was a precursor to what was to become my walking clinic in the future. We walked for three hours until my leg felt like it was going to fall off. I later discovered I had damaged cartilage in my knee.

I examined an old blind woman with very high blood pressure. She had no idea of her age but I figured she was about as old as my mother, and when I finished speaking to her I felt so drawn that I hugged her. Somehow, despite great difficulty, she got off the bed and began dancing; slowly at first and then gently and smoothly, she praised and worshipped God. I held her close and did the same and soon we were both dancing. She was crying and I was not far off. I will remember her until the day I die.

There were several other older women suffering malnutrition. A staple of the Ugandan diet is *matoke*, which is a meal based on plantains, a green fruit that grows in bunches like dessert bananas. The skin is peeled and then the plantain is steamed in a cooking pot lined with leaves from the plant over a charcoal stove. It is then mashed and served with ground peanut sauce poured over it. *Matoke* is almost pure carbohydrate and is lovely. The other staple food is *posho*, which is corn meal and cheaper than *matoke*.

As I was leaving, I noticed a young girl and asked Recheal to ask her how old she was and if she was pregnant – she explained she was fifteen and her baby was due next week. She had been raped by someone in authority on the council – an 'old man' – so there had apparently been no point in calling the police. She was so small and thin that her baby would have only weighed a kilogram. This tiny girl should still have been at school, innocent and with a future. I arranged for her to see Edward, who later referred her to Mulago. I knew the baby would not survive but I prayed she would.

That week I visited Mulago Hospital to see several people I had referred there and was reminded of how sparse the facilities and care was. Stephen was suffering cancer and needed treatment; he had been in hospital for three weeks waiting for radiotherapy with his mother caring for him and sleeping on a mat on the floor under his bed. I paid someone to push him in a wheelchair to radiotherapy when it started because his mother couldn't. I then found Moses, the little boy who had been found in the pit latrine. He was doing well but no-one had come forward to foster or adopt him, so he stayed in limbo in hospital. At least he had some new clothes to wear courtesy of Australian donors, plus a long cuddle from *mzungu* Judy.

The lack of pharmaceuticals was chronic in every health facility I visited. There were some drugs available over the counter in Kampala but they were out of the price range of most of those suffering. I seemed to be visiting a chemist almost daily to buy something for someone. The clinics and hospitals had some medicine but I was worried about how these were stored and monitored. Even the most basic drugs we take for granted in Australia are hard to come by in Uganda, and I felt that any impact I was to have in the future must involve bringing medicines in from Australia.

I made an appointment with the Uganda Drug Authority and quickly discovered that bringing pharmaceuticals into this country was not easy. The government had strict guidelines, in part a reaction to other countries dumping their out-of-date medications here which then had to be destroyed. Given the strict controls, in hindsight it would appear to be quite a miracle that I sailed through the airport with my first bundle of medication donated by OPAL. I suggested to the authorities that such heavy restrictions could make it too difficult for me to bring any useful medicines back in the future. The Ugandan Drug Authority told me it would require law changes if I was to import drugs from Australia so I decided instead to purchase what I could in Uganda. Eventually I found where to buy medications in Uganda although they were often poor quality.

That day I returned home to Frank and Michele's to a familiar pattern. Halfway through a shower the water stopped running and then the power went off. As I ventured into the kitchen wearing a dressing gown, I was surprised by a complete stranger who walked in looking for Frank. We then heard the news that three people living nearby had died of AIDS in the past twenty-four hours, and five more in the village of Nakulabye. Life in Uganda just seemed so cheap and it upset me. It wasn't that I wanted to hear that it would all be alright because it knew that it wouldn't: it was awful and hopeless and I wondered if I was making any difference at all.

Chapter Seven

As my round of patients grew, I effectively developed a pastoral routine of stopping off at the clinic or the Mulago Hospital to check on patients I had referred there. I wanted to make sure they had been seen by medical staff, had food to eat and if they wanted me to pray with them I did – I had quickly learned that in Uganda prayer is a major part of life, with prayers held before and after meetings and certainly before every meal no matter how basic.

Afterwards I headed into the slums. Although it was physically tiring and my knee ached, I often found myself feeling humbled by the humanity. One teenage boy was described to me as having been 'down with the fever' for eight or so years. He was beautiful but he didn't speak and had the appearance of cerebral palsy. Cared for in a dark room, mostly by his grandmother, he had sores on both his hips and was lying on the floor with an old shirt as bedding. I dressed his wounds and spent an hour showing his grandmother how to clean his teeth and exercise his fingers, and to take him outside to hear the birds, feel the breeze on his face and be stimulated by his surroundings.

Nearby lived a beautiful twenty-five-year old named Rita. She was tall and thin with tight black curly hair common to Ugandans. She had high cheek bones and beautiful dark eyes that lit up even though she was terminally ill with AIDS. She had been admitted to Mulago but received almost no treatment and so was home again. She had lost an enormous amount of weight in one week and said she knew she was dying, so I began advising her on palliative care. She had a four-year-old daughter Bridget, a gorgeous little girl who was bright and bubbly. I feared she might have AIDS like her mother.

Rita's sister Robina was taking good care of her and I was told that all other members of their family were either dead from AIDS or far away. I found out later that there was another sister Margaret who lived in a village away from Kampala. Robina had children although I never met them. She did not look anything like her sister. Her skin was lighter in colour which suggested they had different fathers.

As we walked back from Rita's house I heard a child screaming. A three-year-old girl had all but severed her little toe, but the suturing was beyond me because tendons were involved. I wrapped her foot up and brought the girl to the clinic, wrote a referral and gave her carer, a girl who looked about thirteen, money to get to Mulago Hospital. The mother of the child was herself in hospital. I wondered how well she would be treated, because if the suturing wasn't done properly she would probably lose the toe.

I had been away from home for nearly three months. As the end of my time in Uganda approached, I thought more and more of home. I missed Allan beyond description and hung out for emails, letters or occasional calls from him. The only chance I had to speak to my children was the twenty-four hours that I had spent at the Sheraton Hotel. Sending letters was difficult and frustrating. There is no mail delivery in Uganda and all mail has to be accessed at the post office. There are thousands of post office boxes and it can take many weeks for a letter to get through and be sorted. There were no internet cafés, so if I wanted to send an email I had to write it out in longhand and then pay an office girl to type it up and send it. Not the best way to tell your family that you miss them. One day I walked a couple of kilometres from the clinic into town to the African Craft Village to buy something special for Allan. I found a beautiful piece, an elephant and her baby carved out of a single piece of ebony. It was quite heavy, so I bought a special bag so I could carry it on the flight home as hand luggage.

Michele agreed to video a day in my life in Kampala, including the clinic and Nakulabye, so those at home could see what it was like. We spent the morning visiting patients and the afternoon in the clinic. Edward was consulting from an old armchair while I dispensed medication, weighed babies and did anything else that came up. When I felt myself starting to run out of energy, Michele found me a can of lemon squash to get a quick shot of sugar and stay upright. We finally ate lunch at

3.30 pm and then Edward and I visited more patients on a walking clinic. Rita, who I had met a few days before, had a severe chest infection, enlarged spleen, no appetite, nausea, diarrhoea, headache and dizziness. Edward told me she didn't have to die yet and organised some medication she could afford.

During my final days we returned to the Wall of Fire Church to see the new room built for the two *jajas* (the Luganda word for older women). I gave Beth a new dress and she looked gorgeous in it. While we were there, we treated heaps of children and their mums for worms. Among them was a small boy known as Smiley, who had the most dreadful rotting feet from chiggers, a harvest mite that attaches to the feet, lays larvae and often brings disease with it. Pastor Matthew from the church had rescued him from a rubbish tip.

In my final week Frank and Michele decided we should be tourists for a day so we all piled in the Pajero and drove out of Kampala. We took Beth and Gerard out of school which made them very excited. They had ice-cream for the first time on our visit to Jinja on the shores of Lake Victoria, almost one hundred kilometres north-east of Kampala. Best known as being the source of the Nile, it was a beautiful spot. I took a photo for Allan of a statue of Gandhi in a small memorial garden where some of his ashes were scattered; we had visited Gandhi's house in Mumbai and his life impressed us greatly. The Bujagali Falls near Jinja were more like large rapids, but I spotted a little cottage near the water and again thought of Allan. We had often spoken about renovating a little cottage overlooking the water and I imagined us there. On the drive home, Beth slept with her head in my lap.

It was very difficult saying goodbye to Rita because I knew it would be the last time I would see her, and I felt quite emotional farewelling Tewo too. We had become good friends and I had given her a start in becoming financially independent by helping her start her small business selling second-hand clothes. She was slowly recovering from her grief over William's death and the business was going well. I gave Jeffrey's wife, Jennifer, money to pay the school fees for her daughter; she was now yet another widow of the AIDS epidemic and there was so little assistance for these women. A fledgling support group for widows had started meeting in Najjanankumbi to socialise and visit the elderly abandoned women in the village, taking them small gifts such as pieces of soap. They included me in their discussions about how best to take care of these people and I knew I wanted to support them somehow in the future.

Although I had many questions in my head about any commitment to working in Uganda, my time ended with a spiritual exclamation mark. I had brought about 200 t-shirts with me from Australia, donated by friends and members of my church. After a discussion with Alice at the Florence Nightingale Clinic, we decided to stage a children's party there and distribute the shirts then along with some bags of jelly beans that my daughter, Fiona, had sent. I didn't quite anticipate what excitement such a basic event would cause.

Michele and I arrived at the clinic an hour early and people were already waiting. By ten o'clock there were more than 250 people outside, including many whom Alice called 'very important'. I sent out for more biscuits and popcorn and we made cordial. The t-shirts from home were handed out, cameras snapped, speeches made and I was interviewed, prayed for and wept over. I had to make a speech in response and was finding it very emotional and difficult, and then an extraordinary thing happened. I picked up Fred, the baby who had come into the clinic with pneumonia three months ago. As he fell asleep in my arms, I leant back against the wall of the clinic for support, watching all the excitement going on around me and my memory was triggered. I had been so focused on getting to Uganda, and so busy once I arrived, that I had all but forgotten about being marooned in the outback and the picture in my mind of me holding a baby and being surrounded by children. While there had been many times over the last few months when I had held a baby in my arms, this was the first time I felt that everything was exactly as it should be, that the vision had been fulfilled. It is hard to explain, but I truly felt that God was smiling and his spirit was upon me.

As a farewell gift I had bought some new equipment for the Florence Nightingale Clinic, including a sphygmomanometer (an instrument for measuring blood pressure in the arteries), buckets, a paraffin pressure lantern, umbilical cord clamps, scissors and bowls so that two babies could be delivered safely at once. I had also been showered in gifts and prayers myself, but the best present came on my last day in the clinic when a little boy was born. I was asked to name him so I called him Gillies, after our minister at home.

I was told I had planted the seeds here and that they would grow, but I also knew a good gardener returns to do the weeding. My mind was spinning with what the next phase of this would be. What could be done from Australia to help the people of Nakulabye?

Chapter Eight

THUNDER CRASHED AND HEAVY rain fell the morning I left Uganda. I was exhausted and emotional, and my suitcase felt like it weighed a tonne. Michele had invited Edward and Rose for supper on my last night and Rose gave me a beautiful woven basket. As we drove to the airport I feared I might miss the flight because the rain had left the main road submerged forcing us to travel down a series of slippery back roads. I flew first to Lusaka in Zambia and then on to my scheduled stopover in Harare, where I soaked in the hotel bath. When I spoke to Allan my eyes filled with tears. I always knew we loved each other totally and with respect, but the depth of this love was a revelation.

Before I left Uganda I had been determined to gather as much information about the community as I could. During meetings with community leaders in Najjanankumbi and Nakulabye I catalogued population, employment, common and prevalent diseases, literacy levels, incidence of malaria and HIV/AIDS, and the numbers of babies receiving immunisation. I wasn't sure what to do with all this information or how it was possible for me to make any difference, but as Allan often said, 'Do your best and let God do the rest.'

As I killed time in the airport lounge in Harare a couple of days later, my thoughts turned to my eldest son, David, who flies for Qantas and who I knew was on an overseas flight somewhere. Once on board, I settled in with my book, ready for the long flight to Perth, when David walked up the aisle. After my initial astonishment, he suggested I follow him to the flight deck where I sat behind the captain. The take-off was delayed for a few minutes while antelopes were cleared off the runway. After we were in the air, David sat with me for half an hour at my new seat upstairs in business class; it was such a precious gift after three months away. I found out later that everyone we knew in Australia was in on this wonderful surprise. I slept all the way home after a delicious glass of champagne. Allan was at the airport along with Gillies and Wendy and some other friends. I fell into Allan's arms. Later I gave him the statue of the elephant and he loved it, gently turning it over in his hands to see how it was crafted. On the drive home he admitted to being lonely while I was away, and so we decided to get a dog. Annie the lovely golden Labrador joined us soon afterwards.

Coming back to Australia was a shock. In Uganda there are no big supermarkets, but back home I would walk into Woolworths or Coles and find so many different products, with dozens of varieties ... and ice-cream. On my first visit you rarely found ice-cream in any shops in Uganda, and here in Australia there were so many different varieties. The wealth of Australia almost seemed obscene compared with the poverty of Africa.

This was the first instalment of the price paid for being in Africa: not a financial cost, but an emotional one. Another, of course, was that while I was away, I missed Allan desperately along with our children and grandchildren, my sister, Mum and friends. I was quite sure many people didn't understand what I was doing or why, but Allan did and his call was to let me go and deal with any consequences at home alone. But probably the greatest price was my complete exhaustion; the emotional drain of coping with injustice, poverty, disease, greed and corruption took some time to overcome. I had several sessions with Gillies to work through my thoughts and emotions. I found him a source of both inspiration and common sense. It was refreshing to find someone who didn't continually tell me how brave I was or what a saint I was.

It was difficult to catch up with our children. Due to their careers they lived a long way from Adelaide, requiring a plane trip or long drive to visit. Fiona was now in the UK so the best we could do was long phone calls. Career opportunities had led her overseas and we accepted that but it didn't stop us missing her. David was often overseas with Qantas while Peter was often on the move with the army.

I slowly slipped back into my routine of cooking and caravan trips. For the end of the millennium we camped with my cousin Trudy and her husband in the Adelaide Hills. We frequently went on camping trips together. We decorated the trees with banners and balloons, had a gourmet meal and toasted the new century before it got so cold we tucked into bed before midnight arrived.

I stayed in touch with Edward and Michele via email although the connections with Uganda were erratic. Neither of them had their own computer and so relied on friends or internet cafés in the city.

I was welcomed back to church and asked to talk about my experiences. I stood up and spoke for a few moments then, as I finished, suddenly said, 'And of course I am going back next year.' I was a bit stunned when this came out of my mouth, because I hadn't discussed it at all with Allan and had always said there would be only one trip to Africa. I looked across the room at Allan and was surprised to see him smiling back at me. Edward was excited when he heard I was returning. I asked Michele if she could find out about accommodation in the city so I could be closer to the clinic. Her house was an hour's travel each way. She emailed back suggesting a hostel that was walking distance from the clinic.

The church began fundraising so I could assist the community and clinic at Nakulabye. I wasn't sure just how but a few ideas started to filter through. For one thing, this time I did not ask for t-shirts but rather some money so that I could employ someone to buy them in the local market, thereby putting money into the community.

I had left Africa bruised and battered emotionally, and coming home to Australia had made me confused and upset at times. But being back in Allan's company had rested and healed me. In October 1999 he organised my flights and in March 2000 I returned to Uganda.

Chapter Nine

I WAS A MIX of emotions on the flight. It was six months since I had left and I ached to renew the intense relationships I had formed in Africa. But there was also a part of me that worried about the reception I would receive. I was wary of being taken for granted and wasn't sure if I would meet my own expectations of making a difference somehow. A lot of people back home seemed to think I was working miracles. The church had given $4000 for me to use in Nakulabye and I didn't want to let them down. All my life I had known exactly what I was doing, where I was heading and what I wanted to achieve. I was forthright and focused and, at times, too outspoken. But now I truly believed that God was remoulding me and in doing so cracking a hard shell I had built over many years. I still was unsure exactly what my path would be, and this frightened me. To be honest, part of me yearned for an easier road to walk.

My arrival at Entebbe was so joyful. Frank, Michele and Hannah Heyward were there, along with Edward and his youngest daughter Olivia. I sailed through customs again and was re-immersed in the smells, heat and noise of the bustling city. Amid the chaotic traffic, a young boy ran behind the wheels of a large truck that was belching black smoke while grinding its way up a gentle hill. His job was to put rocks behind the wheels to stop the truck sliding back.

I booked into the Namirembe Resource Centre Hostel, a facility run by the Church of Uganda for girls attending the nearby secondary school. They house about sixty girls with six single rooms for short-term visitors. It's popular with Western travellers and workers because it is safe, clean and cheap, but the Pentecostal church across the road seemed to have almost non-stop singing and praying from about five o'clock on Saturday afternoon and finally ending twenty-four hours later. The noise was excessive and intrusive, but requests to lower their amplification in the past seemed to have been ignored. The packs of dogs that also howled and barked to accompany the worship made such a racket that one night I prayed the dogs would be struck dead. Then I thought God wouldn't be happy with that so I revised the prayer and asked for an outbreak of canine laryngitis.

Eventually I met Anthony, the young pastor from the Pentecostal church over the road. He in turn introduced me to a woman named Judy Howe, a missionary from Toronto who was also staying at the hostel. She had an infected foot which I treated, and during the conversation she mentioned she was moving into a little house and asked if I wanted to share it with her. I said I would prefer to stay at the hostel because it was close to the clinic, thinking I would need to know her a little better before making such a commitment.

Edward took me on a tour of his hospital, which he hoped to complete in three months. This seemed rather optimistic: the bricklaying was finished and the roof was on but he had run out of money, and there were no doors, plumbing, electrical wiring or windows. He also had no idea where his equipment and furniture was going to come from. I had been given a microscope in Australia for Edward and he was very impressed with it. He had a tiny laboratory in his old hospital and this would enable him to do more blood tests and diagnoses.

My first day back at the Florence Nightingale Clinic in Nakulabye started in an unusually quiet way because Alice was away. Suddenly it burst into life when children came running from everywhere and showered me with love, running their fingers through my hair and holding onto me tightly. Cheeky little Thomas from next door refused to let go; he was very thin and I feared he might have AIDS. He quickly became my shadow, following me as I consulted. I handed out some sweets and promised to return the next day to check them all out. When I did there was a second outpouring of joy from the children and mothers. One woman sang while others chatted and laughed. Some of the little ones looked plump and gorgeous, while others were clearly not thriving.

Robina, Rita's sister and carer, came into the clinic looking thin and pale in the final stages of AIDS; I hadn't realised the previous year that she was also infected. She told me that Rita had died and that she sent me her love as she slipped away. Afterwards her brother ransacked the house and stole what money she had, and she was to be evicted from the room she had been renting. Unfortunately, in Uganda this callous act of looting after someone has died is very common. Robina asked me to visit, and the next day I found her being looked after by her sister Margaret, who had moved back from her village up country to be near Robina. I paid the A$100 Robina owed in back rent and explained it was a gift from people in Australia. I never had any problem using the money this way because it had been given to me to use where I saw need. I knew my church family would not want to see this woman evicted from her tiny room while she was dying of AIDS.

I felt such sadness. The people of Uganda were dying all around me and there was so little I could do. During the day I would steel myself for the sights and sounds of unstoppable suffering, and in the evenings I would pray but most often just felt powerless and sad. In this state I wasn't eating properly. Every time I tried to eat a larger meal I would feel sick or bloated, so instead I snacked on biscuits, two-minute noodles and my trusty jar of Vegemite.

I found solace at All Saints' Cathedral where one Sunday morning the service seemed designed for me. All Saints is in the city of Kampala on top of a hill overlooking the business district and it holds services in English. I had happened upon it almost by chance when I was catching a bus to another church one Sunday. A car stopped to offer me a lift. Inside was a family on their way to the Cathedral which became a comforting place for me. The first hymn was 'Great is Thy Faithfulness', which came as an answer to the anguished prayers I uttered at night. The sermon was based on Exodus 3 and 4, where God directs Moses via the burning bush. I decided I would no longer worry why God hadn't called someone better qualified or more holy than me here. The reality was I felt that God had chosen me and I had said yes. On the way home I bought a large bag of fresh fruit to eat, which left me feeling spiritually and physically in much better shape. All Saints was to become a regular place of worship where I found peace and renewal.

My first meeting with Alice didn't convince me the Florence Nightingale Clinic was being managed any better than last time. Alice had a wonderful heart but no mind for money, and many documents recording the clinic operations were pure fiction. One day while waiting at the Nsambya hospital I saw Agatha, the nurse from Nkumba – the clinic by Lake Victoria which I had visited with Edward and Alice. Alice visited this clinic from time to time as part of her work with the Florence Nightingale Clinic. Agatha told me Alice had just sacked her. When I later asked Alice about this she said Agatha had been stealing money and 'other things'. I had no way of knowing if this was true or not, but the more I dealt with Alice, the more concerned I became about the transparency of the operation. Honesty and accountability had always been cornerstones of my work and I felt that I couldn't work somewhere where that was secondary. I was learning fast that I would only find out the right answer if I asked the right question.

In addition, I had growing fears about the basics of the way the clinic was being run. One day I found tablets in a container marked 'dexamethasone', which is used quite freely in Uganda for severe inflammatory conditions, and so dispensed them as such. I immediately realised by looking at them they were not what the label said. Thankfully it turned out they were only paracetamol, but they could have been something that could kill a child. I also discovered that Alice had been using clean but unsterile needles for injections, an enormous malpractice in a country so rife with HIV. A nurse in Australia would never use anything that was unsterile. I was so angry about this dangerous lack of standards that I had to walk out of the clinic for the rest of the day. This didn't seem to bother Alice at all.

Life at the hostel was always unpredictable. The water went off for two days without explanation, so showering became a very basic experience with a twenty-litre container of water, a bowl and a coffee cup in the cubicle. Outside the cubicle was an electric hot water jug, and the trick was to get the temperature and the amount right to tip over your head – especially difficult when your hair needed a wash.

Although it was noisy, the hostel provided an opportunity to mix with a small section of the expatriate population of Uganda.

Along with Judy (before she moved into her cottage) there was Julie, a lawyer from the United States, Jenny, a doctor from the UK, and Venestre, an economist from Burundi. Several times, Julie, Judy and I went out shopping together or for a meal, and often on the way home we would buy fruit and make an enormous salad back at the hostel for dinner. We also discovered a superb local drink made of crushed sugar cane juice and ginger. After Judy moved into her cottage we christened her new barbecue: I bought a Nile perch as long as my arm and grilled it along with potatoes, eggplant, onions and mango.

Frank and Michele Heyward had written to me in Australia about a gorgeous four-year-old orphan called Suzan. Her mother had died in childbirth and her father was killed in the war in Rwanda, so Suzan was being raised by her grandfather in a village outside Kampala. As a toddler she had been badly burnt when she fell over a charcoal cooking pot and now had horrendous keloid scars to one arm, all of her trunk and her right upper leg. Keloid scarring is hard and irregular and will sometimes form after an injury. It is quite prevalent in Uganda and often has the appearance of a thick, coiled rope. Suzan could not stand up straight because the worst of the scarring was in her right groin, and this contracted and pulled her down. If tapped, the scarring on her chest made a loud hollow noise.

After hearing from the Heywards, I was able to raise a few hundred dollars in Australia before I left in the hope that Suzan could have surgery to release her scarring so that she could stand upright. Suzan was now an orphan and had been placed in a boarding school on the outskirts of Kampala to escape the poverty and harshness of village life. It isn't unusual for children in Uganda to go to boarding school at a very young age if there is money to pay for it. When I visited I gave her a doll and a dress from 'Mama Fiona' – my daughter had decided to sponsor her schooling. She sat on my knee and hugged the doll. The matron said they all loved her and she was very bright.

Early on this visit to Uganda, I had read in the paper that a team of Dutch plastic surgeons and staff were visiting Kampala. They came regularly and operated at the St Francis Hospital at Nsambya, a privately operated Christian hospital. I took Suzan along in the hope they could see her, but I feared there would be too many cases and told myself it was unlikely. My fears were increased when we arrived and saw hundreds of people waiting in a line, many with gross deformities. But to my surprise the doctors saw Suzan and booked her in for surgery the following day. She hated every minute of the whole process, screaming and clinging to me because she was terrified of hospitals and doctors due to the painful treatment she'd received after the accident.

The day after her surgery, Edward and I went to visit Suzan in hospital but found her outside the building at the latrine – Edward gave her carer a swift lecture on hygiene and infection. I was responsible for Suzan's admission and her expenses and had raised money in Australia for just this type of situation. I discovered from the staff that they intended to discharge her the following day, so I paid for an extra week in hospital, some new clothes and a potty so the carer wouldn't take her outside again. When I sat down on her bed, Suzan clung tightly to me but wouldn't speak. I sang some nursery rhymes and the little darling slipped straight off to sleep.

Suzan had hope for the future because she was getting an education and appropriate medical care, but so often in Uganda the opposite is true. Robina was still suffering greatly as her body broke down in the final stages of AIDS. I bought some painkillers from a pharmacy and injected them to give her some relief. The need for medicines of any kind, let alone palliative care drugs, was constant in clinic work. Edward showed me a pharmacy in the city that sold good quality medications, and I bought a lovely woven backpack from a street market which I used to pack them into for the walking clinics.

Often, as we walked through slums and villages, people dressed in rags would silently stretch their hands out toward me from the shadows. Groups of older women, many of them widows, lived in squalor and begged for food. I gave away about forty dollars in tiny amounts, and you would have thought I had been handing out million-dollar cheques. I was aware that this was not the answer to their poverty and need but they were hungry and cold. I was learning the difficult lessons of life here in the slums but it was not in my heart to say go away, starve, stay cold, I cannot help you. I did what I thought was right at the time but was to learn that I could do it differently in years to come. One lady lived in a room less than two metres square, with no windows or even a blanket to lie on at night. Nearby lived a thirty-five-year-old named David, who had gaping, pus-filled wounds from his groin through to the rectum. The condition was most likely caused by syphilis and his quality of life was zero. It was so far beyond my ability to treat him that I found a way to get him to the hospital with a letter asking for help.

About a fortnight after I had arrived, Edward stunned me with the news that his wife, Rose, was in hospital in labour. She is a big woman, but no-one knew she was pregnant aside from Edward – not even their five other children. She gave birth to a two-kilogram baby girl by caesarean section and named her Judy. I was overjoyed at the honour. Edward told me it was a way of 'legalising' my involvement in Uganda. Many days I would slip around to visit Rose at home and have a cuddle of little Judy.

In the weeks that followed the delivery, Rose struggled with a bout of malaria. Edward believed she caught it while giving birth in Mulago Hospital because the hospital has no screens on the windows. Nowhere is safe from the mozzies and, according to the Ugandan Ministry of Health, 95 per cent of the country is exposed to moderate to very high transmission levels of malaria. Another awful statistic in a country that was full of them.

Chapter Ten

EDWARD AND I HAD developed a good working relationship and I admired his accountability and honesty. He had invited me to work at the Busabala Road Hospital and so I started a walking clinic each Wednesday while remaining at Nakulabye for the other four days. The Hospital was set in Najjanankumbi, a slum village similar to Nakulabye. I was always accompanied by two or three widows who would take me around to visit the various patients and along the way teach me local customs, culture and language. I enjoyed interacting with the widows and the people in the community. Busabala Road teems with humanity. Little road side stalls sell fruit and vegetables while tiny shops with iron bars over the windows to prevent robberies sell tea, sugar or flour. Along this road there is also the best *japarti* stall I know and we would often stop for one on our walk. A *japarti* is like a bread wrap cooked on a hot charcoal stove. They are delicious just as they are but sometimes when I was at the hostel I would buy one from the local trader and fill it with avocado, tomato and onion.

I had been back in Uganda now for six weeks and began to realise that if I was to do something on a permanent basis it was going to be here in Najjanankumbi and not with Alice at the Florence Nightingale Clinic.

Edward spoke to me about some spare land next to his hospital and the possibility of developing an HIV/AIDS clinic there. It was exactly the same thought I had already been entertaining. I enjoyed Edward's company and admired his work. He was passionate about helping his people and I knew we could work well together We could set up a clinic under strict protocols, where anyone would feel comfortable coming for advice, education or treatment. After realising our shared goals, my discussion with Edward also encouraged me to go a step further: I realised I would need to set up an organisation so I could make my own decisions and collect my own information about Uganda and Ugandans. It was a turning point for me.

These thoughts swirling around in my head had to take a back seat to the daily needs of the people of Kampala. At the clinic one morning, Robina's sister Margaret came in with a huge abdominal mass. I feared that, like her sister, she too was slowly dying of AIDS. After I arranged for her to see a doctor, another woman arrived asking me if I would take care of her children when she died. She seemed to think that perhaps I could take her children back to Australia with me and I had to gently tell her that that was not possible. There seemed such a need for an organisation to deal with the orphans who were such a vulnerable result of the AIDS epidemic.

I found a certain resignation to the disease among young people. They didn't seem to care that they had AIDS and showed almost no emotion in discussing it. It made my heart ache because they didn't expect to live and so had no hope. At times I wished some would die quickly so that they would stop suffering, but at other times I knew their lives could be extended with better care and treatment.

As I watched Robina suffer I grew to hate AIDS. I hated the sicknesses that it caused, the suffering and the despair. In a country teeming with life, I found these prolonged stages of death senseless. I hated too that I was unable to help and the frustration that brought. I couldn't see why God didn't just gather these people quickly to him rather than allowing them to continue in agony.

I eventually took Robina to Mulago Hospital where I said goodbye to this beautiful young woman. In less than twenty-four hours she was dead. Alice and I went to pay our condolences to Margaret and when we arrived I was startled to see a coffin already outside the door. It was crudely made of pine and lined with a cotton cloth, the wood was still tacky from the varnish. Robina's body was inside the house on a mattress on the floor, covered with a cloth. The room was crowded with women while the men hung around the door and the coffin. I sat on the floor beside Robina's body along with the women and we all wept for the loss of this beautiful woman. It became apparent that the burial couldn't take place because they didn't have enough money. Margaret had only half of the A$50 needed, and so my final act for Robina was to pay the rest of her burial costs. Afterwards I arranged for Margaret to be tested for AIDS but expected that she was already well advanced. People told me the level of HIV infection in the Ugandan community was falling, but I only saw the results of people who had been infected years before and were dying. Robina's death haunted me. It often came into my mind when I least expected it, and mixed with the grief was the guilt of not having done enough to help. I wrote to Allan and Gillies about it and hoped the feeling that I had let her down would subside.

One day on a walking clinic in Najjanankumbi I came across an example of how the disease has stripped out generations. A man named Anthony, who neighbours said was eighty-eight years old, was caring for six great-grandchildren aged between three and ten. I found the room they lived in almost unbelievable. It had no window and was only large enough to fit one single bed and a small child's bed. The old man slept on the small bed and the six children squeezed themselves onto the other. During the day he carried twenty-litre cans of water for people in his neighbourhood to earn money to feed the children. The widows had formed a small group at the hospital so they could visit needy people in their community but they had no money to supply anything. With money from my church I purchased blankets to replace the one Anthony was using, which looked like a mechanic's oily rag. We made arrangements with Edward at the hospital to keep *posho* and beans for Anthony to have access to.

Another time a very sick baby arrived at the Nakulabye clinic suffering from malaria and measles. The child was filthy because the mother thought her child shouldn't be washed if he had measles, a common misunderstanding. In addition to treatment, mama got a lesson in basic hygiene and I was reminded again of why education is such an important part of improving health. It was difficult to explain the need for cleanliness in a place like Nakulabye, which was so filthy. Everywhere you walked were horrible smells, excreta, used condoms and plastic bags. It was not unusual to see a small child walking around with a razor blade in their hands because adults used them to cut their nails and then discarded them. I explained to mothers it was a good health investment to buy water (at this time of year, twenty litres cost five cents) and to wash their children and their clothes to prevent illness. Very few houses had tap water connected so water had to be bought for everything. In addition to basic hygiene, I stressed the importance of boiling their water before drinking it.

So many illnesses were symptoms of poverty, filth, overcrowding and malnutrition. Tuberculosis, for example, is one of the top ten killers in the developing world, with three million deaths and ten million new cases each year. The bugs that cause TB are inhaled and, while a healthy person is able to keep them under control, when the body's immune system is weakened by HIV tuberculosis can spread to every organ in the body. Treatment involves a number of expensive drugs that need to be taken over six months.

Lifting people out of poverty is as much a health as a social or economic issue. At the clinic, more and more people approached looking for handouts. Women with babies would ask where I lived so they could come around and become friends. At times it was irritating, but I understood their need and thought I would do the same if the positions were reversed.

I still had money that my church had given to use within the community and I wanted to involve the women of Nakulabye in deciding how it could be used. I wanted them to tell me of their needs rather than me giving them my Australian point of view. Alice mobilised them into attending a meeting and we were encouraged when about fifty women arrived. This was the first time I seriously looked at a financial scheme. There was excitement about the possibility of using small loans for a community piggery or to open a restaurant. The women believed it would cost about A$1000 to set up either so I offered to follow it up with UGAFORD, a local organisation which offers small loans. After the meeting a group of drummers performed and someone tied a grass skirt around my waist. Soon over a hundred people were watching and they went bananas when I joined in the dancing. After catching my breath, a baby was placed in my arms – it was Grace, a newborn baby boy who had been abandoned on a doorstep and was being cared for by the woman who discovered him. I had taken a special interest in him and encouraged this lovely woman. She had a girl aged about six and had been wanting to get pregnant again without success. Little Grace turned out to be a gift for her.

Unfortunately UGAFORD turned out to be a dead end: the widows couldn't even afford the transport to the their office each week to pay their instalments let alone the interest rate being charged. The next step seemed to be using some of the money raised in Australia to start the project. The widows firmed on the idea of opening a restaurant rather than a piggery; their theory was it would be quicker to establish and create a faster cash flow, as a restaurant in Uganda can be as simple as someone cooking and selling food next to a seat and table. There were about twenty women of various ages involved who seemed strong-willed and determined to succeed. They found a building in a good position in Nakulabye. It was a wonderful feeling being able to empower these women to try something positive. With the money they eventually opened this little shop which was part-restaurant, part-Ugandan-style delicatessen. I continued visiting them whenever I was in Nakulabye and the shop is still flourishing.

The widows weren't the only group interested in bettering their prospects. When I was visiting a clinic down near Lake Victoria I met a group of youths (a title which seemed to apply to anyone under thirty-five) to see where I could help. These young people were all unemployed and desperate for a project where they could take on some responsibility and get a little income. We met regularly and in the weeks that followed I donated A$40 to help them start a piggery at Nkumba, about 130 kilometres from Kampala. They bought a boar and two sows, which they named Judy and Matilda. On the day they proudly showed me the porkers, they followed with a song they had composed about helping the poor, starving, lonely and elderly. The young men had such beautiful voices.

After some thought, I came up with an idea for another youth group who came from Nakulabye, stemming from a mixture of wanting to help them have a better life but not wanting to be used as some sort of Australian financial hand-out service. I challenged them to raise the money to buy seventeen pairs of shin pads for their proposed football team. There were so many youths interested, we had enough for two teams. The next part of the challenge was that each team sponsor a child (I already had in mind Grace and Fred). Fred was the beautiful baby who I met on my second day at the clinic. His mama was dying of AIDS and although Fred had been diagnosed with AIDS he was still in relatively good health. If the youth group met the challenge I would cover the cost of their sporting uniforms. I worried that spending such a large amount of money on sporting gear was an indulgence, but it felt like an investment in the community. The group readily agreed to the conditions and committed to taking care of the little ones, visiting their mamas and helping in the children's education.

I met up with Recheal, the clinic nurse who had worked so well alongside me on the last visit. We had a lunch of chicken and chips followed by ice-cream; she said it tasted funny and would have preferred Ugandan food. About to turn twenty-one, Recheal told me of her desire to be an enrolled nurse. As a nurse aide working with Alice she had only had minimal training in the very basics of community nursing.

Over time I had become very fond of Recheal and liked the way she handled the patients who came through the clinic. She was respectful with the mamas and gentle with the babies. I wanted to give her the opportunity to have a better education. After discussing it with Allan via email, we decided to sponsor her.

I arranged for her to enrol at a hospital run by the Church of Uganda at Kiwoko, a two-hour drive north of Kampala. The course took two years and cost about $1000 per year. Recheal cried tears of joy when I agreed to sponsor her training, and Edward committed to being her supervisor. He arranged for her to work at his hospital during her breaks for extra experience and also gave her a sharp lecture in front of a group of people about his expectations. He explained the opportunity she had been given and that she should set a good example, work hard and not get pregnant.

I visited Beth and her mother, Anna-Mary, at their house. They had moved out of the Wall of Fire church and had a tiny room made of mud bricks with a dirt floor, barely big enough for a single bed. The door was kept closed with a bent nail. About ten children suddenly appeared in the room and began singing the evangelical anthem 'My Redeemer Lives'; Beth joined in with great animation and dance moves. I gave Anna-Mary money for a new dress, schoolbag and some food, and for the first time she didn't ask me for anything else. Beth's school books showed she was a good student and her English was improving. She was ecstatic when I gave her a big pink teddy bear.

Since my first visit, there were some improvements in the health of those we saw on walking clinics. The children had responded to having been de-wormed. In Uganda almost everyone has at least one worm or parasite living inside them that can cause harm, and kids can sometimes have more than ten. Many of these worms live inside the bowel and compete for food, but if the child is malnourished they can develop anaemia and swelling of the legs. They become tired and can't study at school and are more likely to succumb to infections. Worms are a big reason why up to half the children under five are underweight and anaemic.

I had been thinking a lot about Edward's suggestion that we develop something on his vacant land. I felt quite sure that my contribution to this country was going to continue although I wasn't sure how. I did feel, however, that it was going to develop into community health care in one form or another. So after a lot of thinking I decided to accept Edward's offer to use the vacant land next to his hospital. My essential idea was to create an AIDS refuge and outreach centre that would also allow referrals to and from Edward's hospital. It could be a place for the elderly to visit and perhaps have a meal. Every walking clinic I went on people would come forward seeking help for relatives or friends with AIDS, so maybe this clinic could be somewhere those people could be brought for assessment and to arrange follow-up nursing care in their homes.

Edward and I visited the other facilities treating HIV/AIDS patients to get some ideas. The United Nations runs a worldwide response to the disease known as UNAIDS, and their operation in Uganda was still small but was soon to expand. The UK-based charity Mildmay also has a centre in Uganda. When Edward and I visited their operation in Kampala it was just two years old and we were stunned by the modern facilities. They offered training as well as palliative outpatient care, but none of this was free.

Visiting the various services gave us ideas but we still only had a plot of land within the grounds of the hospital. Edward was using all his spare cash to finish building his hospital and hadn't begun trying to equip it. We discussed setting up an NGO so money could be raised in Australia to create a health care clinic at Busabala Road. I didn't want it to end up like the Florence Nightingale Clinic .

After the success of the previous year's t-shirt day, we decided to stage the event again at the Nakulabye clinic. This time I paid Tewo, baby William's mother, to buy 130 t-shirts with donated money and we bought 150 bags of popcorn, sweets and cordial. Despite my high hopes, the day was a disaster. More than 200 children of all shapes and sizes appeared and quickly resembled a mob. They screamed, fought and punched each other and could not be controlled. They attacked the bags of popcorn and many were split, contents spilling onto the ground. In total frustration I put half of the t-shirts away and never even brought the sweets out. We decided to save them for when children were brought in for immunisations.

My sadness was added to by the sight of little Fred, brought in by his grandparents because his mother was too sick. After progressing so well last year he had regressed, and was now thin and not thriving. He had AIDS, a chest infection and was also teething. All I could do was give his grandparents some syrup to help with the latter and most minor of his complaints. I decided this would be my last day at the Florence Nightingale Clinic; it was so sad to leave on these terms, but I could no longer be involved. Nothing had improved at the clinic and like my first visit I found working there a constant frustration at poor standards and dishonesty. I realised that as long as I was there Alice would use the situation to her benefit. She had mobilised far too many children for the party and we had had a riot. Earlier Alice had suggested I build a new clinic for them when I suggested erecting a simple shelter for those waiting in line. I found a report had been written about the clinic's success – none of which was true. Alice always needed more and I didn't have it to give. Although I still had a week left in Uganda I decided not to go to the Florence Nightingale Clinic again.

In the final week there was an incident that seemed to reinforce my frustration and powerlessness at being unable to help. I was sitting in my hostel room after supper and as usual there were thousands of cars and trucks lumbering past on the busy road outside. Suddenly there was much noise outside the gates of the hostel. A young man had been hit by a car and soon hundreds of people gathered to see what had happened. There is no ambulance service in Uganda and eventually the police arrived and put the man onto a truck which was driven away to hospital. I felt bad that I hadn't helped in some way, and although there was nothing I could really do, the feeling lingered.

As I was packing my bags and preparing to leave, I reflected that this visit had been nine weeks of love, rejection, frustration, tears and prayers all mixed together. But I now felt certain that the way to make a difference in Uganda was to build on Edward's work at Najjanankumbi. My understanding of myself and my relationship with God had matured, and it seemed okay to fail and not be perfect.

In my final hours before flying out, Alice and I talked through the issues of the clinic. In spite of her many failings Alice is a devout Christian and she asked me to forgive her for lying, which I was happy to do. I told her that I loved her and wanted to continue being her friend but that I couldn't work with the clinic again. My focus was now on a new project. Although I still didn't know what it was going to be I knew that Edward would be involved and that he was the one I could trust. Together we could develop something for the benefit of his fellow Ugandans.

Chapter Eleven

EXHAUSTED AND STILL DISTRESSED by Robina's death and the other harrowing things I'd experienced, I flew to England where Allan was waiting for me. It was a cold, bleak London day but it didn't make any difference to me because we were together again. He was my rock to hold on to and provide comfort. We met up with Allan's brother, John, and his wife, Rosemary, for a short holiday, flying to the Greek island of Rhodes to stay in the tiny village of Lindos, which we had previously visited. It was extremely hot but the evenings were superb, especially while eating at a rooftop taverna.

During the flight home I reflected on my visits to Uganda over the past two years. I felt worn down and frustrated, so much so that I actually considered never returning. What sort of impact was I making anyway? Things were done so very differently. Over the following weeks I came to understand that I was looking at it the wrong way around: rather than searching for what I had changed in Uganda, the real issue was what Uganda had changed in me. I had been through an apprenticeship, and now I understood a little of the country and its people. I just wasn't sure yet what I could do with this knowledge.

I didn't have to wait long for the answer, and with it came a resurgence of energy. Shortly after returning to Adelaide I was contacted by the purchasing officer from my old workplace, Resthaven, asking if I would like some equipment for Uganda. They were rebuilding one of the nursing homes and the CEO, Richard Hearn, wondered if I could use the furniture and equipment that was going to be replaced. Allan and I went to have a look at it and immediately knew we had to have it for Edward's hospital: he didn't have the money to finish building it, let alone equip it. Gillies called him the Noah of Najjanankumbi because he had followed God's brief to build something with no idea what it would be filled with or how.

We went to Westbourne Park Uniting Church for assistance, and the church council agreed to underwrite the cost of a six-metre shipping container to send the equipment to Kampala. As we started collecting from Resthaven, word spread and other hospitals (particularly the Repatriation General Hospital) heard what we were doing and offered surplus equipment. The donations ranged from beds and lockers to intravenous stands and pillows. Someone offered a rarely used autoclave steriliser, worth about $4000, which we accepted with delight and took to the supplier for an overhaul. When we returned to collect it, the manager told us they were concerned about the machine going to Africa as it was one of the best in the state, and if any part broke down it would become useless. With his next breath he offered to donate an extra machine to the project just in case.

So quickly did the amount of equipment grow that suddenly the six-metre container was not big enough and we needed a twelve-metre one. The first time I looked at the steel container I immediately realised its potential: after the equipment had been taken out, it could be converted into a clinic in the grounds of Edward's hospital in Najjanankumbi. It wouldn't take much to cut doors and windows in it, and it would be the perfect adjunct to the hospital services. The Kiwanis Club of Adelaide heard about the plan and offered to pay the $4000 required to buy the container. They also insisted on painting it, and a generous donor provided some special heat-reflective paint so that it would not get so hot inside.

We then started having a serious problem with storage. Initially people from the church were collecting and storing donations at their homes, but reports were coming back that their sheds and even bedrooms were bulging. We went looking for a larger place to store the equipment while we waited for the container to be shipped. It so happened that our local Mitcham City Council was in temporary premises while undergoing rebuilding and had a huge warehouse attached that they didn't need. They gave it to us for as long as we needed at no cost. We finished up with hospital, medical, nursing, dental and educational equipment valued at around $350,000 – enough to fully equip Edward's thirty-bed hospital.

Unbeknown to me, Gillies contacted ABC TV's *7.30 Report* and suggested it might make an interesting story. Soon they were around at our house. They used some of the footage of life in Kampala that Michele Heyward shot before I left and interviewed Anthony Radford, who ran the international health and medicine course, Richard Hearn from Resthaven, and me. I showed a harrowing photo of a boy I had met on the last visit named Ronald who, along with his mother, was dying of AIDS and TB. I said that I didn't expect either of them to be alive when I returned. The TV crew then filmed the warehouse full of equipment and outlined in the story that we were still trying to raise the $7000 needed to ship the container to Africa. The story went to air nationally two days after Christmas, and the response was stunning.

Gillies offered to take any phone calls from viewers that were passed on by the ABC. The first person who rang was from interstate and wanted to know more about the project. Gillies started excitedly talking from a faith perspective but she cut him short, saying she was an atheist. She then said she believed in people working together for good and wanted to send $7000. The next call was from a couple who were Buddhists. They also donated $7000. One woman specifically donated money for education, and later her money was used to complete a school building in a district near the hospital. A businessman from Victoria offered $10,000 to pay for generators; he said he gave the money because he knew every cent would go to Africa. A couple from Queensland offered a donation and two weeks later sent the same amount again. They would continue this fortnightly donation for four years.

In all, Gillies took hundreds of phone calls, more than 150

emails and donations ranging from $10 to $10,000. One particular caller stood out because of his heavy accent: his name was Luigi Quarisa and he rang from his home near Griffith in the New South Wales Riverina asking to talk to me. Gillies explained that he could speak to him about the project, but Luigi insisted on speaking to me. Eventually he revealed that he wanted to give some money but not before meeting me. He was so insistent that Gillies arranged it. A few days later I went to church with Gillies and there we met Luigi, his wife, Mary, and daughter, Lizabeth, who had driven more than 800 kilometres to see me.

We quickly found much in common, despite coming from vastly different backgrounds. Luigi was born in a small village in northern Italy called Castelcucco and migrated to Australia in 1950 as a twenty-year-old. On the voyage he befriended a priest who was returning to missionary work in India. When the boat docked in Colombo, Sri Lanka, Luigi was one of a handful of passengers who went ashore. This brief encounter had a profound impact on him. He realised that although he was poor in Italy (his reason for migrating), he had so much in comparison to the poor of southern Asia. He took a photo of the priest surrounded by local children and carried that picture in his wallet for the rest of his life. When he arrived in Australia, Luigi had a 500-pound debt but that didn't stop him sending his first pay packet to the priest. That was the beginning of a lifelong habit of helping those less fortunate than himself. The Quarisas were big supporters of Mother Theresa's Sisters of Charity and in 1993 travelled to India to witness their work firsthand.

After seeing the story on the *7.30 Report*, Luigi was frustrated that the ABC didn't indicate how donations could be made, and so his daughter, Lizabeth, eventually tracked Gillies down and helped arrange the meeting. Although they were open to giving, Luigi and Mary were wary of charities retaining large portions of donations for administration. After talking for forty minutes about Uganda, Luigi and Mary made a very generous donation. Lizabeth declared she wouldn't miss out and dashed to the car, returning with her own cheque. As they left, Luigi and Mary insisted I promise that when Allan and I were next caravanning we would stop in Griffith for a cuppa. I didn't know it at the time, but it was the beginning of a wonderful friendship.

In the space of a few days we had ten times the amount of money needed to ship the container, and so the scale of plans changed dramatically. Instead of just basically equipping Edward's hospital we could now complete it by paying for mosquito screens, electricity, plumbing and doors.

A week after the story went to air, I was at home with Allan when *The 7.30 Report* rang again. Because of the overwhelming response from viewers they wanted to do another interview, only this time it would be live to air with the fill-in host, George Negus. I hurriedly agreed and within a short time a van pulled into our driveway and technicians began converting Allan's library into a mini studio. Gillies soon arrived to lend support. It was a different experience from the first time around because now I had to look straight at the camera lens and listen to George via a tiny earpiece while surrounded by lights and cables running everywhere. In my ear I could hear the introduction as they replayed part of the story of Ronald and how I had needed to find the money to ship the container. Given the speed with which events had moved since then, it seemed so long ago. Then the interview began.

> **GEORGE NEGUS**: Judy, it's nice to meet you, at least down the line. Apparently since that *7.30 Report* went to air, things have looked up for you, there are a few generous souls up there.
> **JUDY**: Oh, yes. We've been overwhelmed at the generosity of people all around Australia.
>
> **GEORGE NEGUS**: How much money has been flooding into Adelaide since that report appeared?
> **JUDY**: There has been many thousands that have been promised and just today we received quite a large cheque, and there are many more that are coming. They're coming from people I would never have expected had money to give.
>
> **GEORGE NEGUS**: How much money were you after initially?
> **JUDY**: Seven thousand dollars.
>
> **GEORGE NEGUS**: Do you think you've exceeded that?
> **JUDY**: Well and truly.

GEORGE NEGUS: That must make you very happy. I guess that means your plans have now expanded themselves. There are other things that you can do when you get back to Uganda.

JUDY: All I wanted to do was to get the container to Kampala. But now it looks as though we can put on electricity in the hospital. One of the big things you need in Uganda is a safety fence, and that means a very high fence with razor wire around it. I can go ahead now when I get to Uganda and have that put around the whole hospital and what is going to be my clinic, and then from there it means that we will have security inside and I can get my friends out there. They will assist me to plant some crops, we can have some goats and be self-sufficient within the clinic. So I guess our counselling service for people dying of AIDS, education for the mothers and children is going to go ahead. This was my vision and I thought it would take about five years, and it's going to happen a lot sooner.

GEORGE NEGUS: I looked at that original story today and you said at the time that if you could hold one Ugandan baby you felt as though this might make a difference. This is going to make a much bigger difference than that.

JUDY: We can save a lot of Ugandan babies now.

GEORGE NEGUS: I imagine that your friend Edward would be rather pleased to hear this news. Does he know about it?

JUDY: No. He knows the container is coming but I haven't actually said to him that we had been on television. I just felt that I would like to wait a couple of days to see if the money started to come in. So tonight we get on the email and I will be writing to him and I will be telling him what we can do. And in true fashion, Edward will write to me back a letter and he will say, as he starts every letter with, 'I am praising Jesus because of the Australian people and their generosity.'

GEORGE NEGUS: When are you heading off? Have you got that far down the track with your plans?

JUDY: Yes. I am hoping to leave Australia in the first week of April, and I will be gone for three months.

GEORGE NEGUS: All the best, Judy. It's wonderful to talk to you and actually meet you in this strange television way, but all the best to you and your project and your friends in Uganda. We know you are going to make a difference and thanks to all those people out there with big hearts who sent that money.

The response from enthusiastic supporters across the country transformed the scale of the mission. We didn't even have a name so people just started calling it 'The Uganda Project'. Up until now the administrative work had all been carried out in the church office, but rightly our church council thought it essential to segregate the project's finances from that of the church. More than $70,000 had been sent to us and we needed to show all that money was going to Africa. A committee was formed in both Adelaide and Kampala so this rapidly expanding project was run in a consultative and accountable manner. Gillies agreed to chair the Adelaide end and was joined by Allan, Anthony Radford and two church members, Ian Attenborough and Fred Wilson.

Fred helped collect the equipment from Resthaven and confessed to finding the work 'contagiously exciting'. His enthusiasm continued when Gillies asked him to dust off his accounting skills and write receipts for the donations. He soon became a lynch pin in his role as committee treasurer, while his wife, Ailee, became an incredible support and wonderful friend.

Gillies asked Fred to help because he was finding it difficult keeping up with his pastoral work and administer this fast-growing project. He was also dealing with his own personal tragedy as his only son, Nigel, was killed in a car accident outside Brisbane on 10 February, the same day hundreds of supporters gathered for a barbecue celebration at the warehouse. At the memorial service, Gillies asked that donations be made to help Edward's hospital in lieu of flowers, and $3500 was collected and saved for a special purpose.

With the warehouse groaning under twenty-six tonnes of equipment and supplies, we paid professionals to pack the container. They completed in three hours what would have taken us a week, and I'm sure we wouldn't have squeezed everything in. It was packed to within two cardboard thicknesses of the door and I ceremonially placed the last item in – a two-dollar broom.

As well as coordinating the equipment collection, Allan had meticulously noted it for customs purposes. The paperwork was tedious but he knew every screw and bolt in that container. Eventually his list for customs was for 582 items:

30 hospital beds

30 mattresses

31 pillows

30 bed overlays

15 bedside lockers

2 pillow risers

1 small chair overlay

2 bed overhead handgrips

1 cradle

1 nurse's clinic desk and chair

1 bed screen

1 four-drawer steel record cabinet

1 two-drawer steel record cabinet

5 intravenous stands

13 hospital chairs

2 doctor's examination stools

1 doctor's travelling chest

1 doctor's high stool

1 shower stool

1 small four-drawer nurse's cupboard

1 small wooden nurse's locker

6 commode chairs

3 cleaning trolleys

1 doctor's desk and two chairs

1 desk light

2 pick-up sticks for disabled patients

91 walking sticks

27 walking frames

3 support handrails

14 three-wheel walking frames

26 pairs wooden crutches

8 pairs metal crutches

5 metal elbow crutches

8 single wooden crutches

13 wheelchairs

2 urinals

13 bedpans

1 toilet raiser seat

3 medical infra-red heat lamps

2 hot/cold water storage urns

1 hospital trolley/examination bed

19 storage boxes for surgical supplies

1 bed bolster

2 small boxes sun protection hats (for clinic use)

2 small boxes surgical and medical dressings

21 small boxes surgical supplies and dressings

1 small quantity dental instruments

1 small box speculums and syringes

1 woollen overlay for prevention of bed sores

1 piece vinyl & mat for nurse's clinic floor

1 piece shadecloth for nurse's clinic roof

2 padded waiting room seats

1 small whiteboard for medical notes

1 blackboard for medical/nursing training purposes

1 pack toilet paper for clinic use

1 small electric jug for clinic use

1 electric toaster for clinic use

1 hospital water jug

1 small clinic table

7 small boxes of medical/nursing/educational books

1 box of medical and surgical textbooks

1 small box baby clothes/soft toys for clinic

1 small box Bibles and soft toys for hospital children

5 litres therapeutic ultrasound conductor (gel)

1 ultrasound instrument

3 electric autoclave units

1 small folding instrument table

1 X-ray viewer

1 operating theatre table with equipment and steps

1 doctor's examination table with steps

1 operating theatre instrument trolley

2 operating theatre stools

1 patient weighing chair

1 operating theatre anaesthetic machine

2 clinic ceiling ventilators

1 clinic broom

1 door frame and door for clinic

2 windows and frames for clinic

1 radio for clinic

1 clothes airer for clinic
1 fibre light projector
1 laparoscopic machine
2 weighing scales
1 box paint for clinic
1 can external heat reflective paint
hospital bed sheets, draw sheets, blankets, pillow cases, towels and bedcovers

When I saw the final list of equipment I was suddenly overwhelmed at the generosity of so many people and organisations. This was really the moment that the Uganda Australia Christian Outreach (UACO) was born.

Our container was booked to sail eight days later, and Allan and I drove to Port Adelaide to see it go. When we got to the gate of the shipping area there was restricted access, but after Allan explained to the man in charge what we were doing he ordered us into his car and drove us to the dock. Our container had been painted white and was clearly visible on the ship. I had tears in my eyes as it eased into St Vincent Gulf on its way to Uganda. I was soon to follow.

Chapter Twelve

ON THE PLANE FROM London to Kampala, the stewardess asked if I would like a glass of champagne. I asked her for two. I didn't need any Dutch courage but hoped soon to be celebrating. Tucking the two miniature bottles into my luggage, I settled down knowing that somewhere, thousands of metres below in the Indian Ocean, the shipping container was approaching Mombasa in southern Kenya. Edward had told me that my first two years in Uganda were an apprenticeship. Perhaps this time I would deliver more – starting with enough equipment to fill his hospital. And this time I had a real goal: to set up a clinic within the grounds of the hospital and educate the mamas so it would become a community health hub. Each walking clinic would be an opportunity to tell mums about the clinic and how different services would be provided on different days. And deep down I knew that getting the container to the hospital grounds, emptying it and converting it into a clinic would be as much as I could handle.

I arrived in April 2001 at the start of the wet season. Edward, Rose and little Judy welcomed me at Entebbe airport. Judy had weighed less than two kilograms when she was born and still seemed to be catching up. She was now twelve months old and, having never seen a *mzungu* before, she was initially wary but slowly warmed up. That afternoon I showed a video to Edward and Rose of an open day we had at home before packing the container to give Edward an idea of what to expect when it arrived. They called me God's angel and prayed I would have a long life and go straight to heaven when I die. I said I didn't mind when I died but that I just wanted that container to arrive intact.

Within a few days we heard the container had already arrived at Mombasa and was on its way to Nairobi. From there it's a day's drive to the Ugandan border and then on to Kampala, all up an 1100-kilometre journey on the back of a truck. There were plenty of horror stories of shipments being held up for months on end, bribes having to be paid and even containers being looted. In Uganda, palms get greased at almost every official level; it is common for parents to pay teachers bribes to get their kids into university. So Edward called it a miracle from God that the container was moving so quickly. But, as I have learnt, few things are straightforward in Uganda.

I set myself a challenge of learning fifty new Lugandan words per week, but language was no barrier on the first walking clinic. The *jajas* were so excited to see me, they flung their walking sticks (tree branches) to the ground and held onto me instead. Those who could danced around, and women came from everywhere in a gaggle of chatter and laughter. I was thrilled to see some were not pregnant this year. Rita and Flavia from the widows' association came along accompanied by a band of young people called 'lady scouts' which, curiously, included a couple of young men. They had been enlisted to do things for the old people, like cleaning their houses and compounds.

Between all this joyfulness, I was distressed to see one of my old ladies, Bitajuma, in a very poor state. Although blind for years, she was now also paralysed in her right leg, and she was hungry, thirsty, dirty and lying on a wet mattress from her incontinence. The grandson who was supposed to be looking after her was now well on the way with AIDS and even filthier. I arranged a mattress from the hospital with a thick rubber coating for her and some sheets. Her grandson disappeared somewhere and I didn't see him again. Between me and the lady scouts, we promised to visit her regularly.

Anthony was still alive and caring for his six great-grandchildren. Despite being worn down by the years, he continued his slow walks down the hills to bring back jerry cans of drinking water for people who tipped him for the service. Our first clinic had begun in an uplifting way, but by the end I was also weary – it was not just the smells and noise that were familiar but also the sorrow. I headed home to my guesthouse in the heat and stifling humidity. Before it rains in Uganda, the sky is heavy with cloud, and the perspiration just pours off you until you almost beg for the heavens to open.

Mama Jude

I thought I had seen a lot of traumatic things in Africa, but within a week of arriving I was witness to something that will stay in my mind forever. Edward had taken me to see a group of Congolese refugees he was treating. We arrived at a large two-storey house where we met a Catholic priest, Father Michael. He was also a refugee and had been living there for about four years. In this house, including the shed at the back, lived eighty-seven adults and forty children, the youngest being four days old. They were so poor they often went without food for up to three days. They had crossed the border in a desperate attempt to escape the ethnic and civil war that has racked the Democratic Republic of Congo since the mid 1990s. Millions have died through violence and starvation and those who survived have experienced indescribable horrors.

One man called Mane (pronounced *mine*), who looked about thirty-five, was a qualified social worker with an organisation in Congo caring for orphans. After being jailed for resisting government soldiers, Mane said he was flogged with a lash twenty times every morning, twelve times at noon and another twenty times in the evening. He was then told he was being transferred to another jail for execution, but a warden helped him escape. He went home to discover soldiers had raped his wife in front of their children, who were now gone,. He continued to his parent's house and found they had been 'slashed to pieces'. His only option was to escape. He still doesn't know what happened to his children. His face held a look of total despair, like the walking dead. He said he desperately needed to do something, anything, so he had a reason to wake up each morning. There was nothing I could do for him and during the time I was in Uganda I never saw him again.

Edward told all the women and children to come to the clinic for immunisation and education on safe sex, because some of the women were prostituting themselves for food. I had never seen squalor on this scale before, nor stared in the face of anguish and hopelessness such as this. They were three months behind with the rent and threatened with eviction. The only things I could think of to assist was paying the young Congolese men to unpack the container and giving Father Michael food to be given to the refugees.

The container remained in Ugandan customs with no sign of being released. Meanwhile, my own accommodation was causing problems. On arrival I had checked into a guesthouse but became quickly frustrated by the tiny room, which was only two paces wide and four paces long, with no drawers or space to unpack anything. The first night I rolled back the bed covers and discovered a bat in residence. Although it was only the size of a mouse, as it began flapping around and making a noise it seemed to grow to the size of an elephant. I quickly got dressed and went down to reception, then a beautiful young man named Joseph came and removed it while I took out a large tin of insect spray and sent a cloud of pesticide over the room. The power went off but was quickly restored when the manager fired up a particularly noisy generator outside my window. I tried to block it out by listening to some tapes but even the music was drowned out by the thumping noise.

Despite my commitment to bug spray, by morning I found myself covered in bites. I navigated my way through my luggage into the tiny bathroom and listened as fellow guests loudly cleared their throats and hoicked. As I sat on the bed feeling rather desperate, I picked up a note sent by Judy Howe, the Canadian evangelical I met last time, who lived in a sweet cottage with two large alsatians for company, plus a night watchman armed with a bow and arrow. On my last trip Judy had offered to share her house with me. Scratching the bites, looking at my belongings stacked on top of each other and wishing the generator would come back on to drown out the revolting bathroom throat chorus, it suddenly seemed like an offer too good to refuse. I rang, just to tell her I was back, and she shrieked, 'Get ready for at least ten hugs and lots of screaming with delight.'

When we met a few days later, she burst into tears of happiness. I immediately asked if the offer to share her house was still open and she cried some more. I had paid for two weeks in advance at the guesthouse and decided I would see that time out, but as the day went on the itchier I got and the more I yearned for my own space. So later that day I rang to see if I could come straightaway – Judy cried some more. She had been very lonely and having a tough time financially, so the combination of company and shared expenses thrilled her. Edward came to collect me and, as we drove to Judy's house, he told me bats carry mites. I realised what had been the cause of the trouble.

Judy's cottage was brand-new and she had taken a lot of trouble to make it homely. It had a functioning bathroom and a kitchen where I could cook. Financially I was better off than at the hostel or guest house and had more independence too. I was in seventh heaven.

Wednesday, 2 May 2001: the day the container arrived. Edward and I went to the Kampala bond store and checked it was intact, after which came a series of events that, if I didn't know better, I would have believed was a deliberate, systematic test of my patience.

On Monday, Edward told me he thought it would be on the block on Wednesday. Wednesday came and went. On Thursday, customs said signatures were still needed. On Friday, the clearing agent said he was having difficulties and still needed some signatures, but it would be Saturday morning for sure. On Saturday, the agent went to get the final signature but the person who had to sign wasn't at work. On Monday, he got the final signature but as it was four o'clock the bond store wouldn't release it because it was too late for processing. The Ugandan Revenue Authority had to observe the unloading on our site. This didn't happen on Tuesday because it was a public holiday.

Wednesday morning finally arrived and Edward and I drove out to the bond store very early.

A crane delicately lowered the container onto the back of a flat-top truck, which then lurched out of the customs compound into the chaotic traffic. We followed in a car behind and as we moved toward the main road, I was horrified to see the truck suddenly turn left instead of right. I raced ahead and flagged it down, only to be told the driver was going to get fuel. I had to suppress a smirk when I saw across the back of the truck a sign saying: 'Don't follow me am also lost.'

When the container finally arrived at the hospital, the Congolese men worked their hearts out. The only instructions they needed every now and then was *pole em pole*, meaning 'slowly, slowly'. The packing was so good that nothing had been broken on the way. At one stage I feared the worst when representatives from the Ugandan Drug Authority asked for an inspection. I opened the first box and they looked inside, ticked off their paperwork and said that I was obviously a busy woman and they would let me get on with it. TIA – this is Africa.

It was like Christmas as the beds, wheelchairs, walking frames, cradles, crutches, baby clothes, medicines and dressings were unloaded. A camera crew from the Presidential Press Unit at Uganda TV recorded the work, while two women from the Uganda Revenue Authority sat and listed everything that came out. Their only real interest was in the cardboard boxes, and asked to open only one of those: the doctor's bag full of instruments and medical textbooks inside made them happy.

The rooms that had only hours before been concrete shells suddenly looked like hospital wards. Patients who had been lying on old blankets on the floor were eased into beds and could now be moved in wheelchairs. Equipment was stored in cupboards instead of on the floor. I gave a knitted hat and scarf to our night watchman: he was thrilled to know a *jaja* in Australia had made it for him.

The container was practically empty in about two and a half hours, with the exception of the anaesthetic machine and the operating table. I hadn't wanted to unload them until the container was off the truck and solidly on the ground, but I then realised that couldn't happen because they would move when the crane lifted it to its final resting place. So the wonderful Congolese workers climbed up inside the container and lifted this precious equipment out; I was so nervous I couldn't bear to look. It went perfectly, and soon the crane arrived and lifted the container gently onto the concrete foundation that had been prepared for it a few weeks previously. A workman immediately began installing windows and doors on the container as it began its transformation into a clinic.

All of a sudden, people started arriving and a celebration began. The Permanent Private Secretary to President Museveni on Religious Affairs opened with prayers, and Edward made the most beautiful speech of thanks. Then it was my turn. Having no idea that any of this was going to happen, I flew by the seat of my pants and explained that my tears were of happiness, and everyone clapped. During the day a reporter from the *New Vision* newspaper interviewed me and we made every TV news program that evening.

We finally went to Rose and Edward's home for lunch about 3.30 pm. Ugandans do not as a rule show their emotions, but

Rose said that she couldn't say the words that were in her heart. And I could not have got the smile off Edward's face if I had tried! He said he was so excited and overawed by the quality of the equipment that he couldn't sleep that night.

At the end of a very long day, I put on some music, showered and collapsed onto the lounge at my new home. I then remembered the little bottles of bubbly from the plane – now safely stowed in the fridge. Judy and I opened them and made several toasts: to God, then the people of Uganda, and my beautiful Australia.

Chapter Thirteen

EDWARD IS SERIOUSLY POLITICALLY connected in Uganda. He seems to have either been to school with, is related to, or is friends with just about everyone. Often when something was needed he would make a phone call or just mysteriously sort it out. I know he has been approached to run for parliament and he often supports others seeking office.

His connections were confirmed when he collected me one morning looking very smart, as the Ugandans like to say. We were heading to a thanksgiving service for the President's re-election and picked up the President's adviser on religion along the way. Driving north towards Sudan through stunning tropical country and then to Luwero along an incredibly bumpy road, we eventually slowed to less than walking pace as the road became clogged with people passing through security scanners. I was wearing my *gomez* and people started to look and smile at a *mzungu* in their national dress. Once past security we were escorted through a huge covered pavilion, across the front of another raised pavilion and up some steps to be seated in the same area as President Museveni.

Yoweri Museveni is one of three principal characters of Ugandan politics since independence in 1962, a period dominated by tribal rivalries, the others being Milton Obote, who was the country's first prime minister and president, and his notorious former military commander, Idi Amin. Museveni studied politics and economics at university in Tanzania in the 1960s, declaring himself both a born-again Christian and a Marxist. He was working in the intelligence service in 1971 when Idi Amin staged a coup and overthrew Obote's government. Museveni went into exile in Tanzania, returning in 1979 as a senior member of the Uganda National Liberation Front that overthrew Amin's government. As minister of defence he developed strong links with the army. In 1980 an election was held and Museveni's newly formed party, the Uganda Patriotic Movement, did poorly, winning only one seat. Obote's Uganda People's Congress won amid allegations of irregularities that heavily favoured the Lango tribe at the expense of the Buganda. It was in this area around Luwero where Museveni and his supporters then formed what became the National Resistance Army. They suffered greatly at the hands of Obote's troops in what was later known as the 'bush war'. Obote slaughtered thousands and there are 70,000 known skeletons in the Luwero district alone. Amnesty International estimates the Obote regime killed 300,000 civilians and a special memorial in Luwero marks 2000 skulls in a communal grave. Museveni is said to have personally counted them.

In January 1986, Museveni's forces took Kampala and he was sworn in as President. Edward admires them greatly and gave me a video about the formation of the Museveni rebel soldiers who eventually marched on Kampala. I don't think Museveni is without blemish, but he did save the largest tribe (the Buganda, which Edward is a member of) from Obote, who wanted to rid Kampala of them and bring in his tribe (the Lango) from the north. Since then Museveni has won two elections, the last being a few weeks before I arrived when he famously travelled on a *boda-boda* to cast his vote.

Luwero is therefore a hugely significant place for those who suffered for Museveni, and the thanksgiving service was ecumenical to say the least. Catholic, Anglican, Seventh Day Adventist, Muslim and Hindu prayers were all said, and it went on for three hours. While I was mostly enthralled, it did get hot and I was dehydrating. I wanted to go to the loo but I felt conspicuous in my *gomez* so only drank a little and hung on until I got home – eleven hours later. As we all lined up for lunch the heavens opened and it bucketed down. I have no idea what I looked like, with my hair starting to frizz with the rain, my *gomez* being held up around my knees and my ankles sinking into the mud, but it didn't matter. Edward appeared at my side with plates of food and we sheltered in the big pavilion. It reminded me of the Bible story of the loaves and fishes, only on this occasion about 10,000 people were fed for free. The majority of people were very poor so for them to have such a feast was truly magnificent.

As I was leaving, the local women became fascinated with me. Edward translated they thought I had paid them a very big compliment by wearing my *gomez*. The women were laughing and calling out as we got into the car, with me feeling just a bit overwhelmed. And so began the biggest traffic jam I have ever been in; it took us two hours to go two kilometres. As we drove along, men and women called out to me so I started to wave and laugh and talk to them in Luganda – I felt a bit like the Queen.

My second dose of Ugandan politics came a fortnight later at a public function to celebrate President Museveni's re-election. Predictably it began with award-winning traffic snarls, which gave me time to admire the streets bedecked with banners of red, yellow and black along with photos of Museveni and his close friend Colonel Muammar Gaddafi of Libya. Gaddafi is supposed to have given him 5000 rifles during the bush war, and it was this plus help from Tanzania that enabled Museveni to deliver the Ugandans from Obote.

The 10,000 at Luwero was a Sunday school picnic compared to this. Among the VIPs were the heads of state of Sudan, Kenya, Tanzania, Burundi and Rwanda, the Vice-President of South Africa, and a former Nigerian president. There were also delegates from Senegal, Ghana, Zimbabwe, Malawi, Angola, Ethiopia, Eritrea, Mozambique, Congo and Egypt. Gaddafi arrived in a white stretch limousine accompanied by his own ambulance, a bevy of four-wheel drives and his personal guards, all beautiful women with long hair, wearing berets, tight trousers and shirts.

The ceremony went for three hours, including interludes by drummers and dancers. Every time Museveni opened his mouth, thousands screamed and blew whistles. I didn't anticipate the twenty-one-gun salute and Edward laughed heartily when I jumped. To add to my astonishment, two Russian MiGs thundered overhead. I didn't even know Uganda had an air force, but Edward told me there are four planes.

Over the weeks the clinic began to take shape. A vinyl floor was installed, iron roof put on, furniture added and a rainwater tank plumbed. We ordered a generator for the hospital, and its arrival was relief for the health workers who no longer had to worry about blackouts interrupting their work. Later a concrete slab was poured for the clinic verandah and I bought twenty plastic chairs, a rubbish bin, a coiled mat for the floor and a mop. Edward helped pay for a stone wall to be built right around the compound for our safety.

I had always thought it would be wonderful to grow vegetables around the clinic, but the ground proved unsuitable. When Edward bought the property it was effectively a steep hill. This was overcome by bringing in about one hundred truckloads of rubble from the Entebbe road when it was being constructed. Although the resulting ground was so poor in quality we couldn't start a vegetable garden, we eventually were able to grow some *matoke* and some shrubs.

Once everything was in place, the new clinic was tested immediately. The sick or parents with sick children lined up outside when I opened the door at nine and I often wouldn't draw breath until one o'clock. My routine was to quickly go through the women to find out who I could treat and who needed to see Edward. One morning, a woman came in who I had met on a walking clinic. She was painfully thin and had three children with her with another two at home. Her three-month-old and six-year-old were fine, but the eighteen-month-old had a raging temperature, bad cough and dehydration. I treated them all as well as I could for worms, malaria and infections. At the end of the treatment, the woman mentioned that her husband had been away but was returning soon, so she wanted to know about family planning. I paused for a moment and thanked God the word was out. I sent the family to see the nurse, Nora, who worked at the hospital, for a quick lesson in family planning. I gave her a small amount of food to feed the children. After they left I wondered how much difference it would make: how would she feed these little ones and herself next week? I was sure the husband wouldn't stay because he apparently left last time because he couldn't cope with all the children. The woman returned the next week for treatment and asked for money, work and food, but I just couldn't give her any more. It made me feel like the worst kind of person.

One morning Nora came to the clinic loaded down with foodstuffs for a nutrition education session. She was a beautiful woman and her smile and infectious laugh brightened every day. We were worried no-one would come, but there were so many mothers we couldn't have fitted any more. Others drifting in later for immunisations stuck their heads in wanting to learn as well. Nora began her sessions by explaining that they didn't need to eat meat or fish to survive but instead taught about the protein, carbohydrate and vitamin content in all the flours, beans and rice she had brought along. When she asked for questions the floodgates opened, and I eventually had to call an end to the session because the babies were getting fretful and it was time to conduct the clinic.

One of the best things about sharing Judy's house was being able to unload our thoughts at the end of long days, often while cooking up fish or a barbecue. I also introduced her to the joys of an occasional glass of wine. We found a butcher who sold proper lamb and cooked a sort of double lamb loin chop, which we renamed 'spine of lamb'. I was even prepared to put up with the rubbish from the men at the market to buy fresh fruit and vegetables; I hated the harassment, but it's the same for all *mzungus*.

With me now sharing the expenses, Judy was able to afford a few luxuries which she had gone without. Together we sought out occasional escapes. Sometimes I would bring the TV home from the clinic so we could watch videos, and other times we met after work to see a movie. One Friday night we headed off to the theatre to see a strictly amateur production of *The Sound of Music*. The theatre was showing its age, it seemed that the orchestra sometimes played from different pages of music, the scenery was basic and at times the curtain got caught in the stage props, but the cast were wonderful. The von Trapps were various shades of white and black, with the tiniest child being a gorgeous little Ugandan who got the loudest applause at the end of the night. The audience was encouraged to help out by singing along and we had a ball.

Another evening we went to see a visiting American evangelist Joyce Myer. After the service we walked home in the dull street lighting and eventually down the pitch black lane that led to the cottage. We were holding on to each other when I said, 'I wonder where our *askari* (guard) is?' Out of the dark came a whisper, 'I am here.' We heard the voice but couldn't see him, he was in a tree watching out for us.

Ugandans have beautiful laughs and smiles, but you also need a hard edge to survive in this country. One evening I was coming home from work in Edward's car. Out the window I saw what I thought was a dog lying on the road, hit by a car. Then I realised it was a boy. Ben, who was driving, said he had seen the boy fall off the back of a truck. We stopped and, as Ben halted the *boda-boda* drivers and other cars from racing up and down the road, I nursed this precious little person in my arms. He was unconscious but quickly came around and became frightened. Onlookers advised me not to touch him because he was 'dust' – a street kid. We put him in the car and drove to a doctor, whose first question to me was, 'Did you hit him?' I replied that I was the Good Samaritan. His next question was who was going to pay the bill. The boy turned out to be fine. His name was John and he spoke no English. He wasn't a street kid but had been hanging around the streets looking for food or money. I paid for the examination plus a tetanus shot and some paracetamol tablets and walked him back to his home with a note for his mama including my name and number. I didn't hear from them, which I took as a good sign.

The episode underlined a fragility and vulnerability I had been feeling on this third trip. I felt totally responsible for the correct use of the container and contents but even more so for the donations which had been given. There had been so much publicity in Australia I felt a duty to show everyone how their hard work was being put to good use. After a lifetime of achieving and allowing others to rely on me, I just couldn't stop living that way, it was part of who I am. Henri Nouwen described it in his book *The Life of the Beloved* as a life lived in a world which is constantly trying to convince us that the burden is on us to prove that we are worthy of being loved. I see myself reflected in that and wrote this in my journal:

People back home think I am some sort of super woman but I am not. I am weak and very, very ordinary and the load is very, very heavy. I am not too proud of myself at the moment. I just seem to be finding things too hard this year. Perhaps I am getting too old for this. Perhaps it is time for me to quit. Perhaps it is just time for God to find someone else to do this work. It seems that the smallest thing that goes wrong becomes a real hurdle for me. Perhaps I am not praying enough. Perhaps I am not good enough for this. I thought that I knew what brokenness was, but this year God seems to be pushing me further and I wonder why?

That Sunday I caught the bus into town and walked for nearly thirty minutes to All Saints Cathedral for Pentecost. At one stage when we were singing, the clapping got louder and faster until everyone spontaneously joined hands right across the church. It was a beautiful service and I felt refreshed and uplifted.

I may have felt spiritually renewed, but physically I was suffering from a painful knee and ankle, so I shortened the walking clinics and found two widows to assist me. I asked them what the people think of the *mzungu* walking around in Najjanankumbi and they replied that many were suspicious, believing I was there to make money by selling photos in Australia. They also thought anyone who accompanied me was automatically wealthy by association. To counter this whenever there were meetings at the clinic I took pains to explain how UACO was a volunteer organisation and that no-one, including Edward and me, made any money. Although UACO shared the same compound with Edward's hospital the two organisations were separate. It worked well because these people went back to the community and spread the word that I was paying my own way. Eventually it turned right around and they thought I had a wonderful husband who allowed me to leave home to visit them.

Despite this, I found the walking clinics to be some of the most wonderful experiences of my life. Every day I met amazing people who taught me the true meaning of respect, kindess, survival and humility. One incredible individual was Bosco, who had been left paralysed after an accident two years before. Married with three small children, his wife made mats and crocheted baby blankets to sell, but there was little demand for them. He had a wheelchair which was so ancient that it was nothing more than a shower chair on wheels. His legs were covered in badly infected ulcers so I arranged for strong antibiotics and dressings and taught his wife, Aisha, how to apply them. When I returned a week later with a wheelchair from the container shipment, everyone was so excited. His friend jumped over a fence to see what was happening and then wheeled him around to visit others and get the sun on his face again. Aisha took to nursing naturally and did a wonderful job dressing his legs and there was rapid improvement.

Another time I met the most beautiful woman named Queenie, who was thirty-three and dying of AIDS. Her father had three wives and Queenie was one of sixteen children, about half of whom had already died of AIDS. Her brother Dan was looking after about twenty sick members of his family. Queenie was too sick to come to the clinic but I promised to visit regularly.

With the success of the restaurant created from the fledgling micro loan from Australia the widows were determined to create more opportunities. They suggested holding education days for those interested. We were discussing who could be invited to talk when Allan rang from Adelaide to tell me the committee in Adelaide had received several donations and felt the money was best spent completing the hospital. When I hung up and gave

Edward the good news he shouted out, 'Praise God and thank you!' After everyone had gone I spent a few hours going over the spreadsheets. I wanted to make sure everything was financially transparent. This was the first time I had done this sort of accounting but it was important given the amount of money that had been donated by Australians. It became a regular practice. In Uganda I had met some wonderful people, but I had also been manipulated and lied to by professionals.

One mortifying experience involved our sponsored child, Beth. I had recently discovered that, despite paying for private schooling for two years, she finished 101st in a class of 101. I was particularly annoyed because back in Australia I received a letter from her written in English, which clearly someone else had forged because she couldn't read, write or speak English. When I had visited Beth in the past she could only say simple English words like hello and thankyou and so her mother did all the talking for her. She clearly had not advanced. I visited Beth in her house and lined up her mother, Anna–Mary, making it very plain that if she didn't put in some effort her daughter wouldn't ever get a job. Beth was clearly sick and losing weight. Edward diagnosed her with hookworm, which attacks red blood cells and explained why she was feeling lethargic and dizzy. I bought a triple bunk bed so everyone who slept in their one little room could at least get off the floor. Anna-Mary asked me for a new Bible because hers was falling apart, so I gave her one plus money for food and clothes for Beth. As I was leaving she suggested exchanging her shoes for my sandals – she got told.

One day all my frustrations with life in Uganda boiled over, so I directed my negative energy with sandpaper. When the container was being converted into a clinic, workmen had cut spaces for the windows and doors to be fitted but didn't protect the exposed steel in any way, so the humidity had quickly turned the edges rusty. I rubbed down all the surfaces and painted on bright yellow rust-stopping paint. Everyone working at the hospital – nurses, guys building the fence, welders and cleaners alike – was fascinated by the *mzungu*. The painters were paid out all afternoon by Edward, who told them laughingly, 'You should go see the *mzungu* – she will show you how to work.'

My three months in Uganda had flown by and it was nearly time to leave. I told Edward that I would return again the following year. Rita from the widows' association came with me on the walking clinic as I started saying goodbye to my *jajas*. They were so excited with the gifts of vaseline (for their skin), sugar, soap and tea that we brought, but also sad they wouldn't see me for another year. One old woman named Alice Mary asked, 'How can one person love me so much?' It was quite an emotional moment for me. She who had nothing gave me so much.

We visited Queenie and Dan. He had got three members of his extended family to help him and although they were young teenagers I spent time teaching them how to take better care of her. They promised to keep her room clean and bathe her. She was very weak and sick and I feared she would only live for a few more weeks. We came across great-grandfather Anthony, who looked as well as someone who is almost ninety and looking after six small children can. I gave him money for food and told him God had a very special place in heaven reserved for such a kind and good man. I found one woman who was very hungry and another desperately needing a blanket. One of the old women said she would die while I was gone and I wouldn't be there for her funeral.

The widows felt that the biggest problem in Najjanankumbi was the orphans. Every widow I knew in this area had taken in at least one of them, and this often led to a lack of food and space. In the long term there was often not enough money for the children to go to school. We decided to start registering the orphans and also made a register of youths, if for no other reason than to get a better idea of the size of the challenge.

The clinic was now operating almost daily. Mondays and Thursdays were for counselling and advice, Tuesdays for immunisations and health care, and there were plans to begin a functional adult literacy school on Fridays. Wednesdays were set aside for walking clinics. My final immunisation clinic was packed and I was thrilled to see the Congolese refugees there in large numbers. The immunisations came from the Ugandan Department of Health. Afterwards the nurses, Victor and Nora, told me that if the clinic had not been there, many of the refugees' babies would have died. I hadn't thought of that before and it was very sobering.

On my last day there was a final flurry of activity, including Florence Kyamanywa agreeing to work as a part-time social worker at the clinic. She had a degree in social work, was married to a doctor and was a good friend of Edward's. I knew she was a gift after witnessing the respectful way she treated the widows at her first meeting.

Edward's hospital was now fully occupied and operational twenty-four hours per day. If anything, this had extended his vision, and he had plans drawn up to convert the original eight bed hospital into an operating theatre. One of our final actions was to register the project officially with Barclays Bank as the Uganda Australia Christian Outreach (UACO) and open a bank account with a $1000 deposit. This only covered the clinic as Edward kept his hospital accounts separate. Edward pulled some strings to make it happen in hours rather than the usual days and said things were moving at *mzungu* speed. The bank required photos for identification and when I looked at mine I wondered who it was: tired looking, grubby, with no make-up nor a comb through my hair, I looked like an old woman – but one who was excited about the future. I had done everything I could think of for the clinic and hospital.

When I sat down to write in my diary I thought of all that had happened and wondered where the strength had come from. My final entry was brief:

I really am a bit of a mess. I am just going to miss them so much.

Chapter Fourteen

I FLEW FROM UGANDA via England and took the opportunity to visit Fiona. It was my birthday and she gave me a day in a beauty parlour as a present. We had several wonderful days together during which I felt so relaxed and spoilt.

I was only home in Adelaide a few days when Peter, Katrina and the children came to stay. Their family had now increased to two little boys, Michael and Joshua. I was reading them stories at seven o'clock one morning when Allan came in with the horrific news of the attack on the twin towers in New York. I rang my mother and she was genuinely fearful that it was the beginning of the end of the world. I was so grateful I was back in Australia with my family but I did wonder if it would ever be safe to travel again and if I would be able to return to Uganda.

Edward and Florence filed monthly reports to me via email, showing the progress being made. I would then circulate them to the other committee members. UACO continued to evolve with Edward bringing together several people in Uganda to form what he called the Executive. Before I had left I had drawn up an organisational chart so everyone knew the structure of UACO. Edward and I were at the top with Florence in charge of the clinic and reporting to Edward. Edward's accountant, Bukenya, was responsible for managing the funds and then the various projects that had been started and the people involved in them. The walking clinics were continuing each Wednesday with at least two widows being accompanied by a nurse from Edward's hospital. In addition, the lady scouts identified where they could help in practical ways. AIDS counselling had also begun, though in a very small way. It was frustrating because most of the assistance went to those in the final stages who needed nursing care because they hadn't sought assistance earlier. I wanted UACO to help break down the barriers shielding this disease and bring it into the open, but I knew I had to adopt the Ugandan ethos of 'slowly, slowly'. The most vulnerable group as far as HIV went were teenage girls, many of whom were orphans. They were constantly being invited to the clinic to learn how not to become infected.

While the AIDS work moved slowly, Tuesdays was the busiest day with mamas bringing their babies in for immunisation. In addition to this, sessions were held teaching about family planning, basic health care, nutrition and AIDS.

A youth department had developed out of a day originally set aside to deal with men's health issues, with a regular group of about thirty young men now meeting to learn and to help around the clinic. They wanted to know about HIV/AIDS, safe sexual practices, literacy and how to manage small income-generating projects. They even formed their own soccer team, despite not having uniforms or boots. Florence had begun training them to talk to other young people about AIDS. Edward was covering the cost of the youth activity which included paying for transport so they could play other teams, soft drinks and occasionally paying for a little bit of coaching. I started thinking about ways they could generate income for themselves. The question of how to alleviate poverty is a constant in Uganda and other developing countries. It is almost impossible to overcome health issues if people are living a hand-to-mouth existence.

Word of UACO continued to spread. Channel Nine's *A Current Affair* featured a story in July 2001 on the project which included pictures of the arrival of the container and an interview with me. Again viewers rang with financial donations. One young woman in Darwin named Fiona Stanley watched the program and immediately said, 'I am going to go there one day.' Two years later she would indeed arrive in Najjanankumbi and be inspired by the walking clinic, the bravery of the widows and the dedication of Edward and his staff. She wrote that it changed her life forever. Although I have spoken to her on the phone and corresponded via email, unfortunately we have never met.

There was also some unexpected interest from the corporate world when Bonds Australia asked if we would like some excess baby clothes. The label on them had to be altered and they considered it cheaper to write the clothes off than replace the labels. Naturally I couldn't say no and our house was soon inundated with more than 2000 tiny outfits. At the same time we received a lovely donation of 168 soft woollen toys made by Julie Lomax and her band of willing helpers from Redhead in New South Wales who'd heard about UACO and wanted to help.

We discovered the best way to ship the clothing and toys was inside four large, steel drums. We packed the clothes, soft toys plus five pairs of donated second-hand Adelaide Crows football boots for the youths. How I wished that I had twenty pairs. The drums didn't have as smooth a ride to Uganda as the container they were in was 'lost' on the wharf at Mombasa in Kenya for several weeks. After much delay and many discussions with the customs authorities, the drums made their way to Kampala and were released to Edward at the hospital. Each clinic day, Florence was able to distribute clothes to mothers who had nothing for their little ones. Some of the soft toys given out were the first these children had ever had. The donation also helped break down barriers by encouraging new mothers to bring their babies to the clinic. In addition to receiving a clothing handout they could get advice, counselling, education and treatment if required.

While UACO continued to grow in Uganda, I was at home eagerly awaiting news of David and Jodi's first child, due in January 2002. As I prepared for Christmas in my comfortable home my heart wandered to Uganda and the people of Najjanankumbi. They wouldn't be inundated with advertisements for the latest toys or people asking what they wanted for

Christmas. Most of them didn't even have electricity let alone a radio or television.

My anticipation of returning to Africa in March was heightened by Allan's decision to join me for the final fortnight. At last he would be able to meet Edward and see all the work that had gone into making UACO happen.

Donations continued to come in, and it was encouraging that many Australians returned with further donations when they heard of the progress. We started publishing a newsletter three times a year to bring donors up-to-date and explain how their money had been used. Westbourne Park Church paid for the photocopying so the only cost we had was the postage. Fred Wilson largely took responsibility for the production of the newsletter along with all the accounting. The Executive Edward had formed in Uganda made the decisions on budget needs and we gave him the amount he needed. Both Edward and Bukenya managed the funds with total honesty. After the exhaustion and self-doubt I felt leaving last time, I realised I didn't have to carry the weight of this alone. I had friends to help and certainly friends in Uganda could manage. I felt a load was lifting from my shoulders.

On the eve of my return to Uganda, an eight-year-old girl from Clare in South Australia's mid-north gave us a beautiful donation. Melinda Grigg had heard about the children at the clinic and had collected small soft toys as gifts. Some were her own much-loved collection, some were from her friends and some she had bought with her own pocket money. Her family drove to Adelaide to deliver the toys and they were the last thing I packed.

Chapter Fifteen

DURING THE FLIGHT, the clouds parted to reveal a wonderful view of Africa. Lake Victoria was dotted with islands and I could see fishing boats hauling in their catches. I had carried Melinda's large bag of soft toys on as hand luggage and there was no interest in it from customs as I walked through into the arms of Edward, Rose and little Judy. Edward was full of questions: How was the trip? How is Allan? How are the members of our church? How is Reverend Gillies?

I was warmly greeted by staff at the Namirembe Resource Centre Hostel, and the Pentecostal church over the road was still in fine form. Despite mixing with other guests, I felt a bit lonely remembering the previous year when I shared with Judy Howe. Judy had returned to Canada after several years in Uganda; her mother was ageing, and Judy herself had some medical problems which needed specialist care in Canada. She hasn't yet returned to Africa but it is passionately in her heart to do so some day.

Edward brought me up to speed on what had been going on over the past nine months. There had been a few staff changes in the hospital: one nurse was sacked for stealing medication while two others were away at training. Florence was a wonderful administrator and it was a delight to have her monthly reports showing what was being achieved and at what cost.

Edward had renovated his original tiny hospital for educational uses such as meetings and lectures, and maternity was moved from there into the new building. The top floor of the new hospital was not yet ready for patients as there was still some work left to do, but it was useful for meetings and training. It was disappointing to see all the trees and plants the gardener put in last year had been eaten by the goats which roam freely in and out of the grounds. That would stop when we had enough money to have gates installed

The training room upstairs was being used regularly for medical seminars as well as for other community issues, including policing. The only problem was that when large numbers of people packed into the room it quickly became an oven. I bought some fans which were similar to the ones in the clinic, and once installed they made a huge difference.

Although Edward was good at getting things done, even he suffered the perennial frustrations of Uganda, such as people saying they would come to work and not turning up. He also struggled at times to finance the renovations because he was paying about A$1500 per term in school fees for all the children he had taken responsibility for. As they grew older, they needed to go to boarding school. He could, of course, raise more money by increasing his medical charges, but he is committed to bringing health care to all. His patients pay 5000 shillings ($3.50) per night, plus the cost of medication. Other hospitals in Kampala charged more than five times that, and the International Hospital ten times, plus a tax of 17 per cent to cover electricity, water and cleaning. Edward doesn't charge the very poor but, in Robin Hood style, adds 10 per cent on for those who can afford it to make up for those who cannot. He had other business dealings that supplemented his income, including property he owned up country where his ageing father lived. He farmed cattle and *matoke* there and whenever Edward visited him he would return with a car groaning with produce.

It wasn't only the hospital that had been growing. I had got to know the Canadian consul in Uganda and he had instigated the donation of six cows for the widows' association. The women had weekly lectures in animal husbandry and soon were milking their cows, feeding their children and selling off the excess milk to make a little money. UACO financed the building of some sheds so the cows weren't stolen. Following this success, the widows applied to the Canadian consulate for eight in-calf heifers to fill up the sheds. Edward looked all over Uganda for good stock, eventually getting them through a friend whose brother ran a large dairy. They were very good quality, and the anticipation built when they got close to delivering calves. Edward bought two litres of milk each day from one of the widows, who lived closest, for about 1000 shillings (70 cents). The agreement was that the widows pay the project back

5000 shillings each month for their cow, which went into an account for expenses such as artificial insemination, drugs and vet fees. The first female calf born was given to the next widow in line. The male calves were sold when six months old and the money put into the account. The first cowshed I visited was immaculate and the cow's name was Gift, as in a gift from God.

Inevitably, some of the widows who had cows died. When this happened the others agreed to offer a $20 comfort fee to the family. In Uganda, it is very important to be able to bury the dead with dignity and this allowed the death to be dealt with properly.

The youth group had grown to about fifty members. They were getting organised in quite a big way, going out and talking to other youths about HIV/AIDS and life skills. I also noticed that they could teach a lot of others about manners and respect. After the success of the football team, I used a donation from a Westbourne Park church member Mary Matthews to fund a cabbage-growing project and to buy them a volleyball set. This meant the girls as well as the boys could play sport.

The mother of three of the youths died from AIDS, so Florence and Ronnie (chair of the youth group) organised food, firewood and a coffin for the funeral. The family had already lost their father and a nine-year-old child to AIDS. It is the custom to give a donation towards the cost of the burial so UACO gave two bags of cement, the amount required to close the grave.

The lead-up to Easter that week was stifling as the wet season set in, with hot days followed by heavy rain at night. Good Friday was my first chance to return to All Saints Cathedral. The church was full and the service was based on the seven times that Jesus spoke from the Cross. The choir sang 'God So Loved the World' and then later, unaccompanied, 'Nobody Knows the Trouble I've Seen'. They also sang in Luganda, a piece about Peter denying Jesus. All were breathtakingly beautiful and left me feeling very close to God.

The Easter Sunday service was also special with everyone enthusing, 'Jesus is alive! He is risen!' Edward picked me up afterwards and we went to his house for a wonderful Ugandan meal of chicken, *matoke*, *luwombo* (ground peanut sauce with mushrooms cooked slowly in a banana leaf), pumpkin, rice, cabbage, Irish potatoes and sweet potatoes. I gave the family the presents I had brought with me from Australia and they were so excited. When Edward saw his tie, he asked, 'Is it from him?' (meaning Allan). He thought it was very, very fine. Although Edward hadn't met Allan he had enormous respect for him allowing me to come to Africa to work. By Ugandan standards it was a big thing Allan had done.

After lunch, Edward went back to the hospital and the rest of us piled in the car and drove to a resort on the lake not far out of town. It was lovely and cool and many were swimming in the large pool. Rose and I had grown to understand each other well and we had many long conversations about life and occasionally how to deal with men. We were walking back toward the car while the other members of the family were several metres behind us, when a security utility raced past with six men in it, guns drawn. They stopped to push a man and woman into the back with lots of screaming. I grabbed little Judy and we ran out of the way. The man who was thrown into the car was calling out that he was a citizen of the USA, but Rose found out days later that he was armed and the pair were thieves. The car sped off with them on the floor of the ute and the six heavies on top. Such events are accepted in Uganda. Stray bullets have killed innocent people in the past, so we got out of there, fast.

Although I had been in Uganda for a week, Easter Monday was my official welcome back day at UACO, but first I went to Nakulabye to see Alice and little Thomas. I was keen to see the mamas and check if their babies were thriving. As I walked through the slums I could hear some young men calling out, 'Mama Jude is back.' When Alice saw me she went bananas, and then children came from everywhere calling out, '*Mzungu* Judy – she is here.' I had to cuddle twenty children all at once. Thomas was taller and still a little larrikin. Not much had changed and there were still many, many people dying from AIDS. There was also an extraordinary number of newborns.

After a cup of tea, a chapati and some fruit shopping at the market, I headed for Najjanankumbi. My goodness, what a party had been arranged! Everyone involved in UACO was at the clinic, with the exception of the old people who were too infirm to get to the clinic. First of all, everyone started ululating and dancing with me. Then there were items by the orphans, the young women, the young men and the widows. They acted out their life predicaments and how UACO has made a difference. When two little orphan boys sang and danced, I was quite misty eyed, first with sadness and then with joy. The women sang and danced to welcome me and I finished up dancing with them, which gave them more cause for ululating. They kept saying it was not a day for speech making, but somehow the speeches flowed. In response I brought greetings from the church and my husband, and they went berserk when they heard Allan was coming to meet them in a few weeks.

The next morning Edward and I worked in the clinic seeing the refugees, who were excited to see us too. The children had grown so much and more had been born. I saw one who was just twenty-three hours old, so I took the opportunity to speak to the parents about family planning. The refugees' problems were still the same and all because of their circumstances. Father Michael said there were now sixty-two adults and sixty-seven children living in the house.

Days in the clinic were hard and we often worked five-hour stints, only stopping for a drink of water. The weather was oppressive and cooling rains were rare and only at night. Women and children often waited for hours outside the clinic in the blazing sun as the verandah was too small, so we used UACO funds to extend it which made an enormous difference to everyone's comfort. UACO, through donations from Australia, paid for gates to be built at the compound, which made Edward ecstatic. Only a few days before someone had tried to break into the maternity ward so we added barbed wire around the top of the fence.

The first walking clinic was wonderful, seeing all my *jajas* and meeting some new ones. Some had died in the past year, but it was so exciting to see Bosco standing out of his wheelchair and walking a few steps. We organised a walking frame so he could get around his little room a bit better.

There were lots of children roaming the streets of Najjanankumbi; they should have been at school but there was no money for fees. Lots of the little ones had colds and runny noses. I found it difficult walking up and down the hills in Najjanankumbi as my hip started aching and I was feeling the full effects of the humidity, but the reception from the people enthused me. Florence had bought soap and vaseline which we handed out along with sugar. Bosco said sugar was the best thing anyone could give him.

One of my old, old women named Sisi saw me from a distance through the door of her house. She had badly swollen legs and could only just walk, was quite dirty and her house was in a state. In spite of all my best attempts at persuasion, she refused to bathe. She said she was too weak to do anything, but her feet had dirt on them from when she had been digging in her garden. I explained to the widows that sometimes we just have to respect the wishes of a person to live the sort of life they do. Sisi said she had not always been like this, and that when she was younger she helped to raise the *kabaka* (king). We gave her a bar of soap in hope.

The workload started taking its toll and my hip now hurt all the time. I couldn't sit for very long and it hurt to lie on my left side. Edward gave me some anti-inflammatory capsules but they

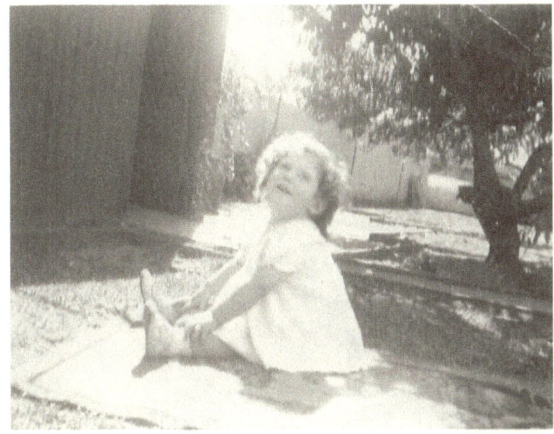

Me, aged 18 months, in Adelaide.

With Dad – a beautiful human being who I never heard complain about his debilitating illness.

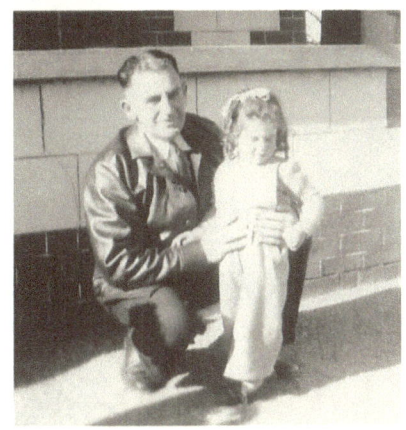

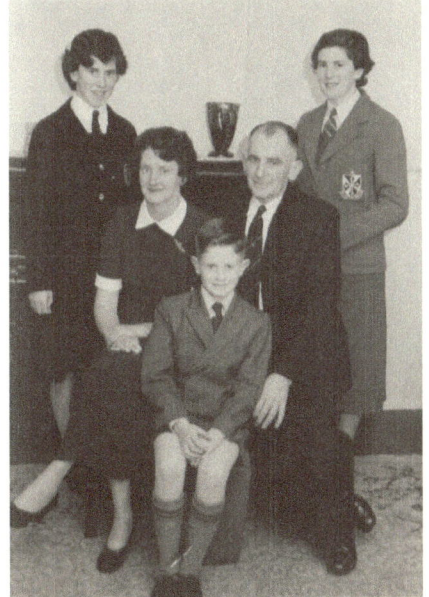

The family at Nangwarry in 1957. I am top left, Elaine on the right, Mum, Dad and Robert in front.

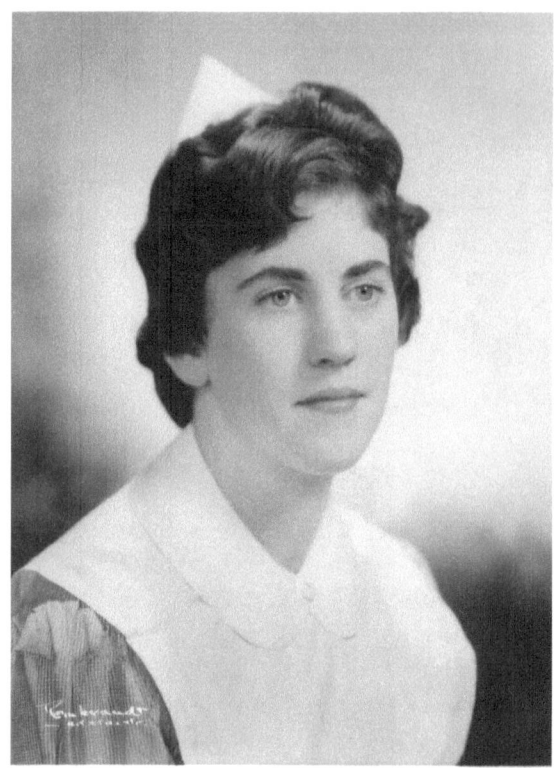

I began my career as a very green young nurse at the Royal Adelaide Hospital in 1961.

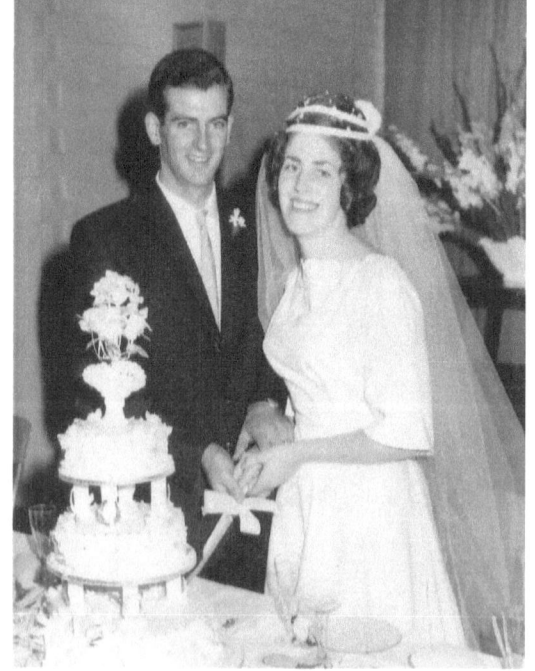

Wedding Day, 22 February 1965.

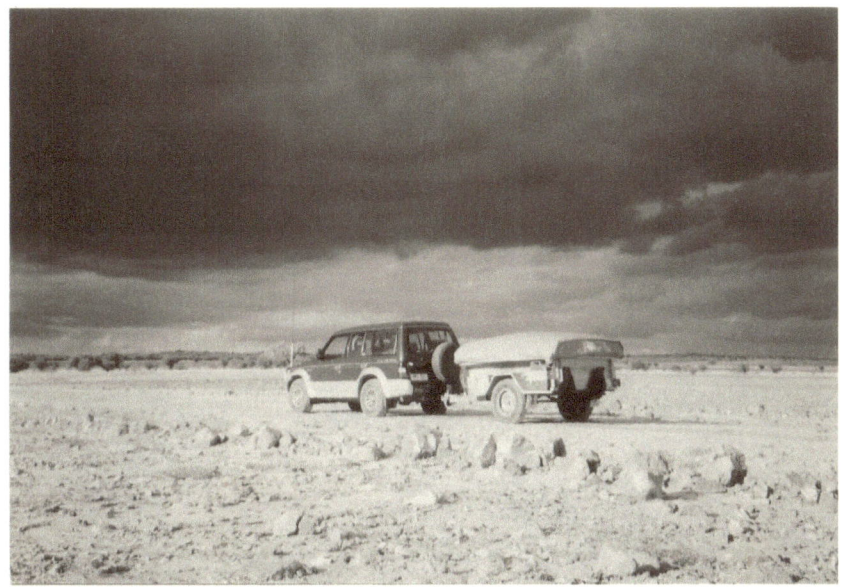

What I call my postcard from heaven. We were stranded by floods on the Strzelecki Track in outback South Australia. It was an experience that changed the direction of my life.

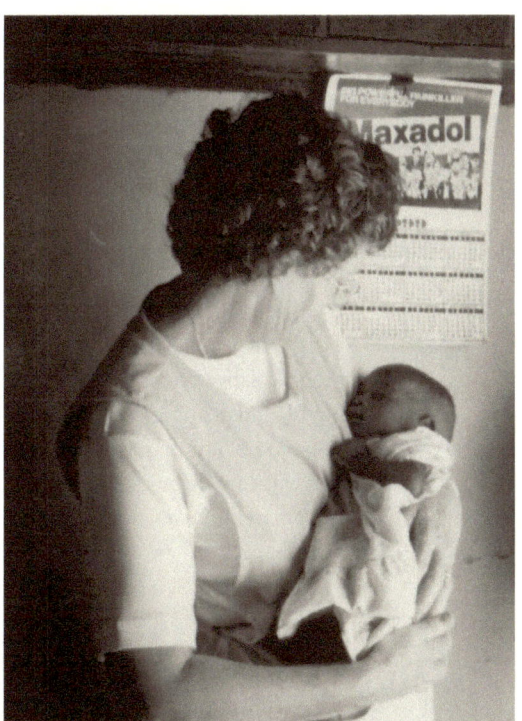

Freddie was brought into the Nakulabye clinic with pneumonia in 1999. I treated him often and he captured my heart. Both he and his mother were HIV positive and died of AIDS.

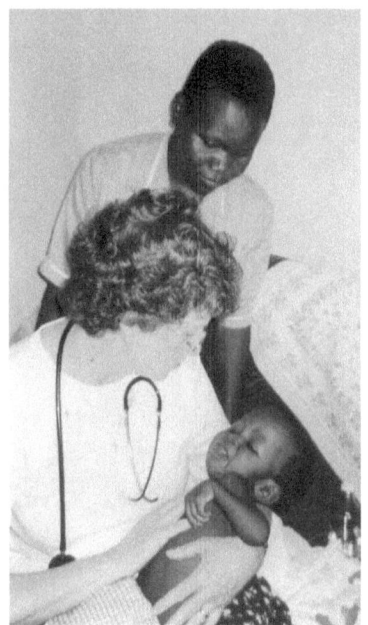

William is ten months old and weighs 3.5 kilograms – this is why I was called to Uganda.

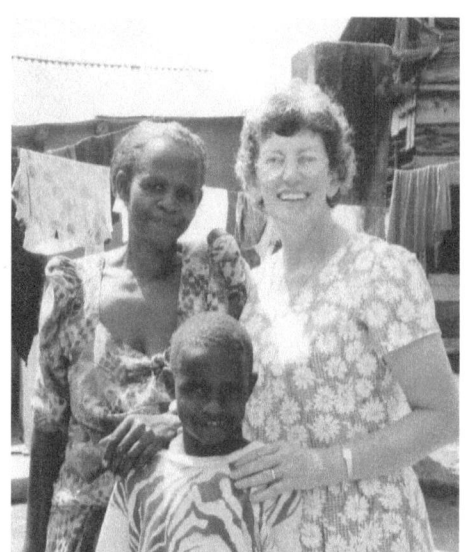

With Anna-Mary and Beth.

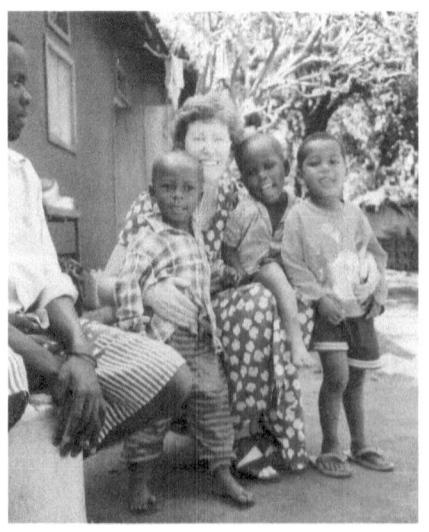

At the Nakulabye clinic where I did my Ugandan apprenticeship. In the centre is Thomas, who shouted out one day when I arrived 'Mama Jude loves me'. It was true.

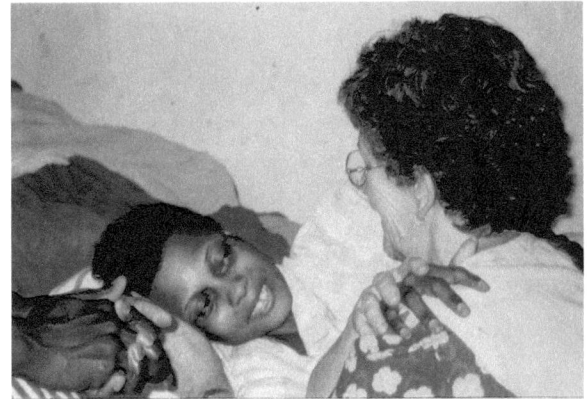

Saying goodbye to Rita, who died of AIDS a few days after this was taken. I grew to hate the disease and what it did to beautiful people.

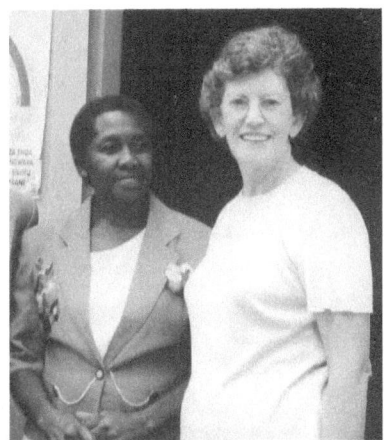

With Alice Zalawango, who ran the Florence Nightingale Clinic at Nakulabye, a slum area of Kampala.

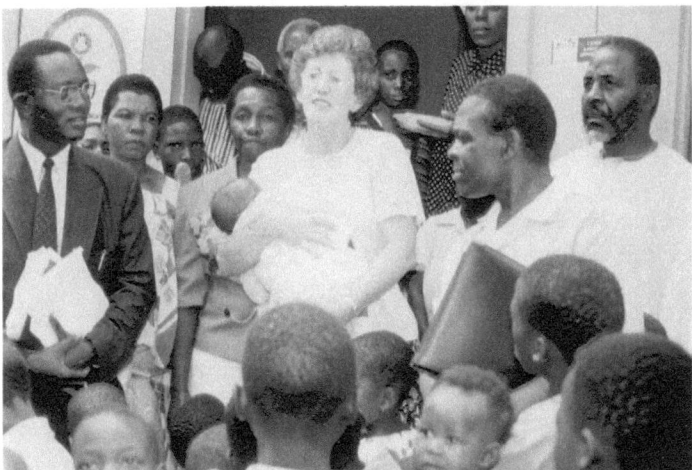

My final day at the Nakulabye clinic, holding a baby in my arms and surrounded by children – the vision that had brought me to Africa was fulfilled. Alice Zalawango is behind my right shoulder.

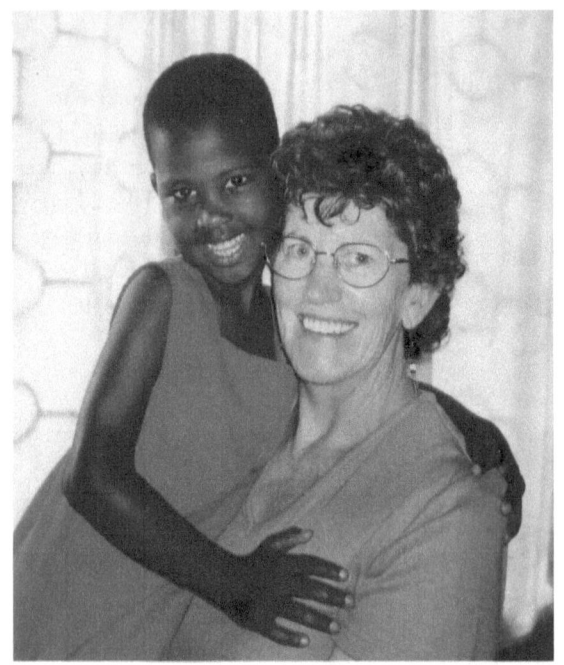

Suzan was badly burnt when she fell into a charcoal fire as a toddler. We were able to arrange treatment and surgery, but she needs ongoing care.

Anthony with four of the six great-grandchildren he looks after. All the generations in between have been wiped out by AIDS. He earns money by carting water.

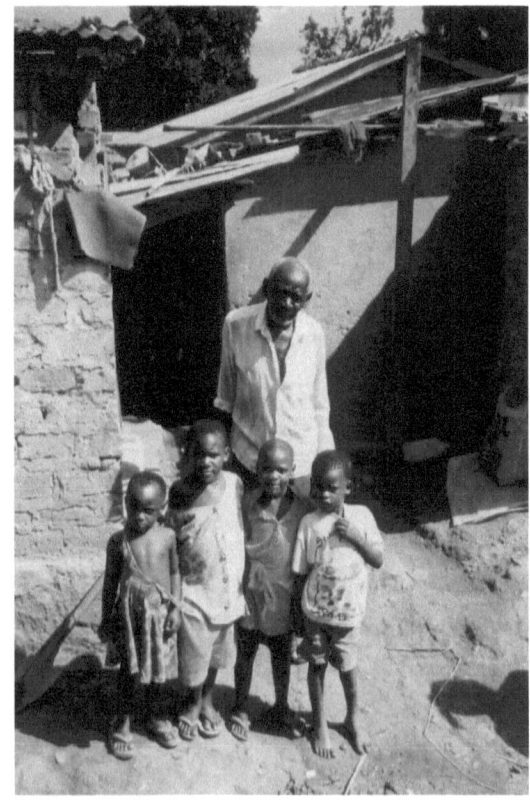

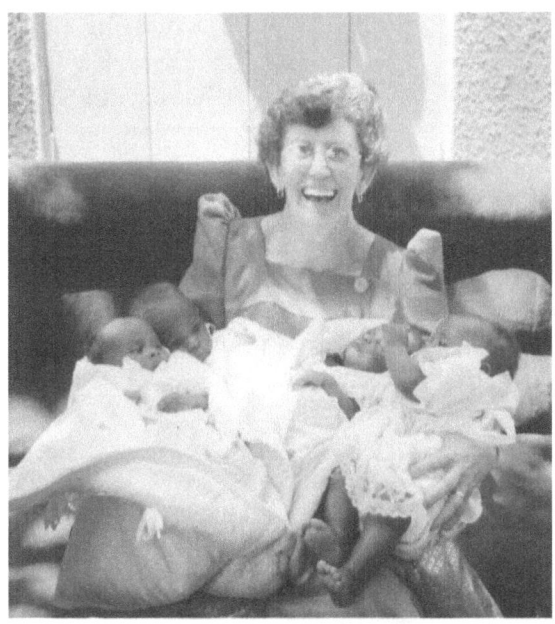

On the last day of my first visit I was asked to name a newborn baby. I chose to call him Gillies. He was one of four baptised that day and was a beautiful reminder of life regenerating amid so much death.

Florence and Ronald, who both succumbed to AIDS.

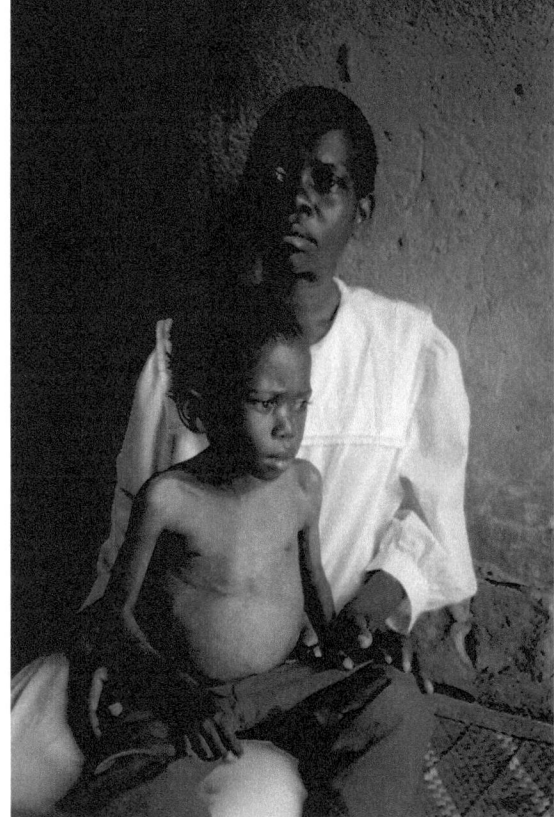

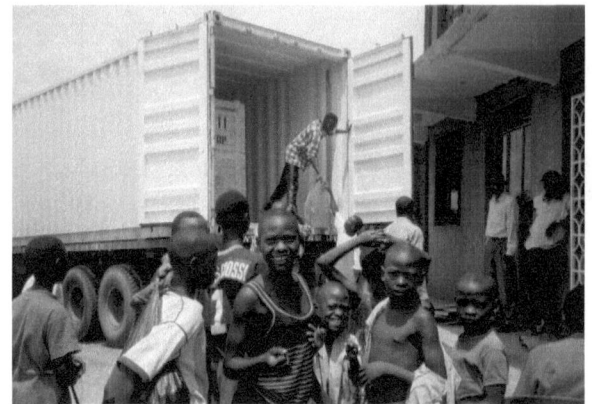

The container arriving with 26 tonnes of medical equipment and supplies donated from Australia. It was the first of three major shipments that fitted out Edward's hospital.

With Dr Edward Ssembatya the day the first container arrived in 2001. I will never forget the look on his face as the equipment for his hospital was unloaded.

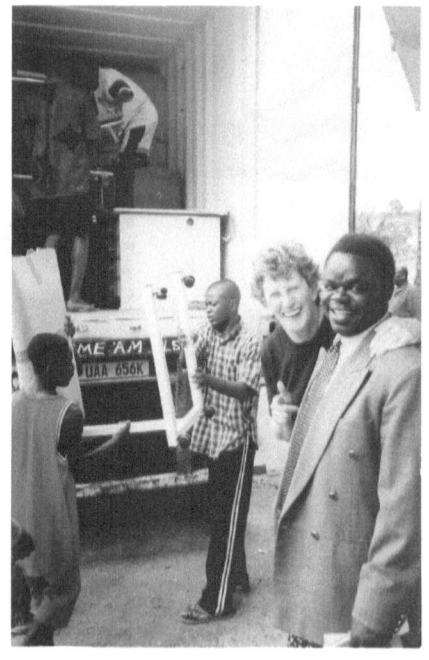

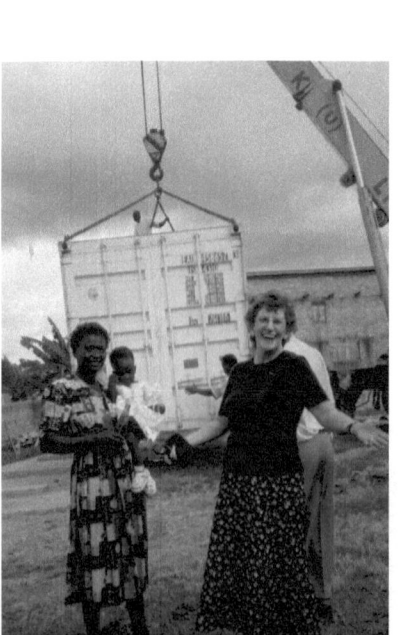

The first container to arrive is placed in position. Here I am with Nurse Recheal, who is holding Edward's youngest child, Judy.

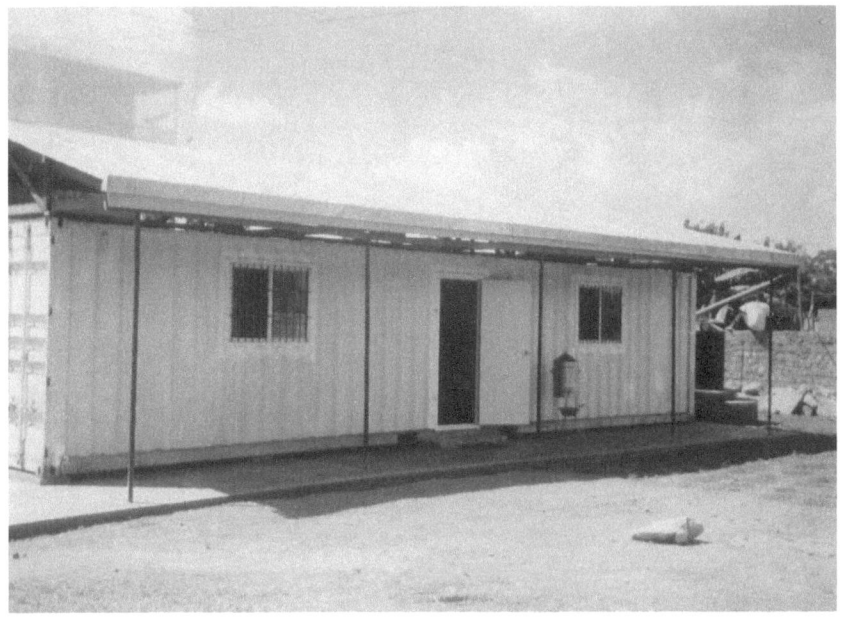

After being emptied, the shipping container was converted into a health clinic on the hospital grounds.

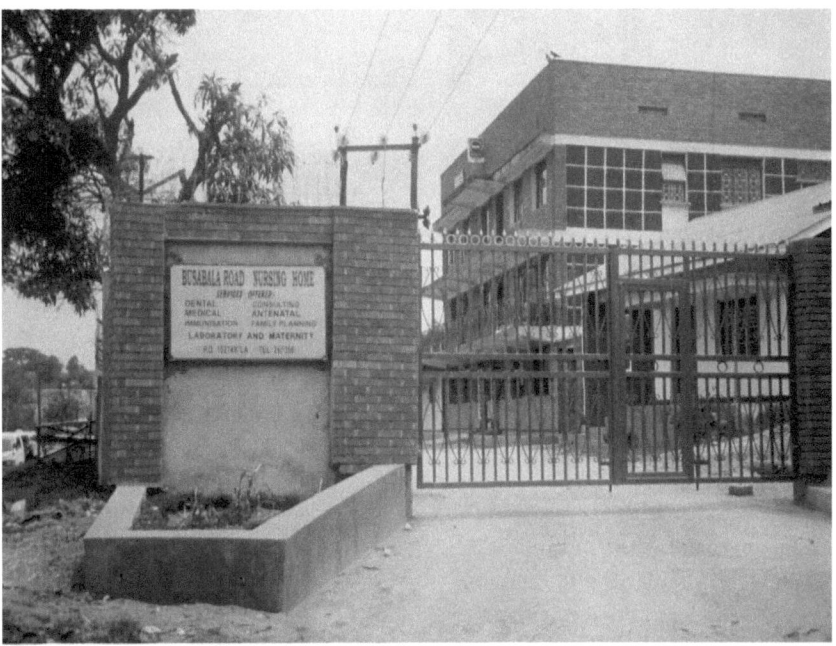

Busabala Road Hospital and Clinic, which was built by Edward Ssembatya, using his own money.

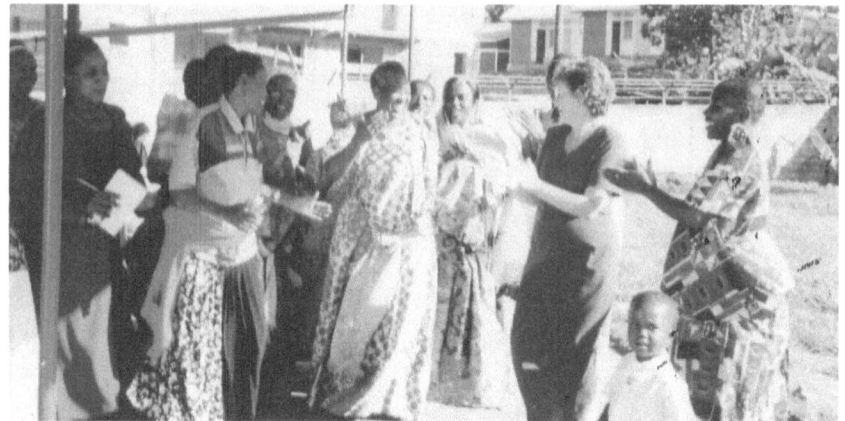

Dancing with the AIDS widows on the verandah of the clinic. Although originally a primary health care centre, the clinic has become a focus of community life.

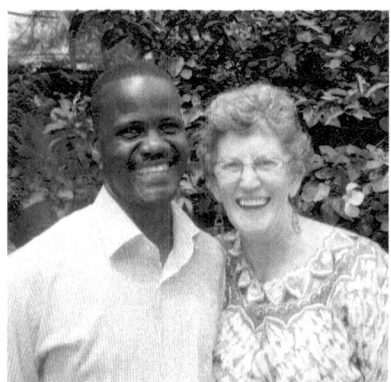

Bukenya is a brilliant, honest accountant who makes sure every shilling is accounted for.

With Edward and my husband, Allan, in front of the clinic built from the shipping container.

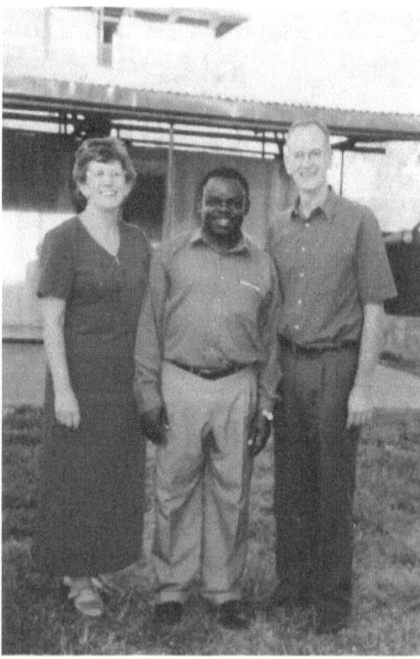

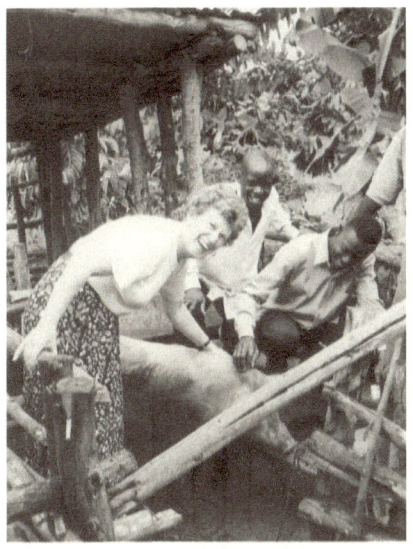

Little did I know that my experience with pigs in the Adelaide Hills would later be important in Uganda. Many small loans were used by widows and young people to buy pigs and a thriving business began.

One of the widows, Ruth, has proved quite an entrepreneur. With her first micro-loan she had a tap plumbed and sold water to neighbours. Since then she has added a chicken farm and extended her house for renting.

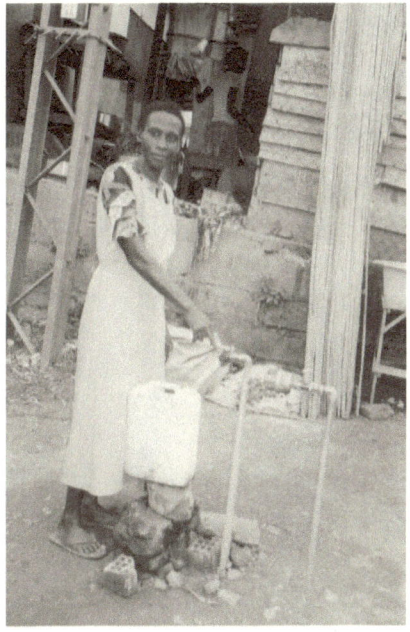

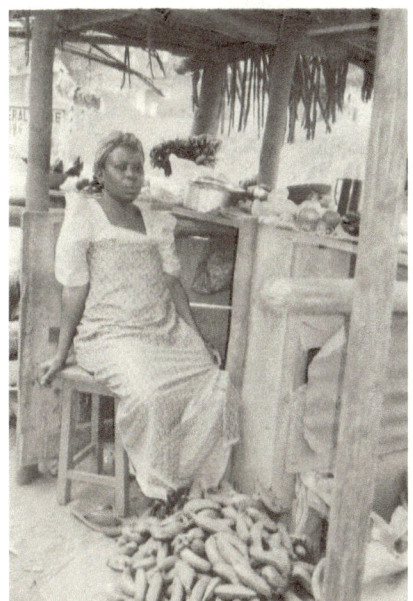

The micro-loans have had an extraordinary effect on people's lives, allowing women to start businesses selling charcoal or, as shown here, *matoke* (made from plantain). They can then afford to feed and educate their children.

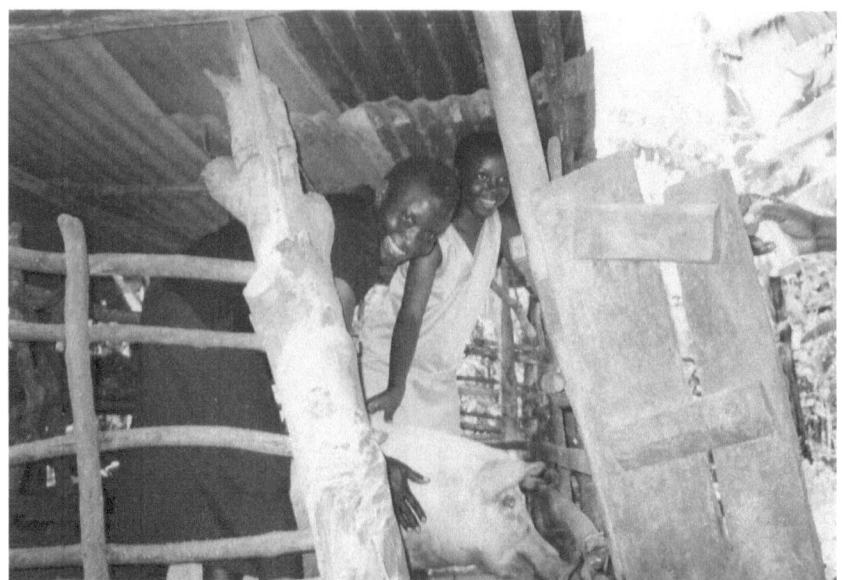

Jane and her daughter Patricia with their pig, bought with a micro-loan. Jane's husband had been a successful trader until he was murdered in Tanzania. Pig farming provides her with a chance to earn some money again.

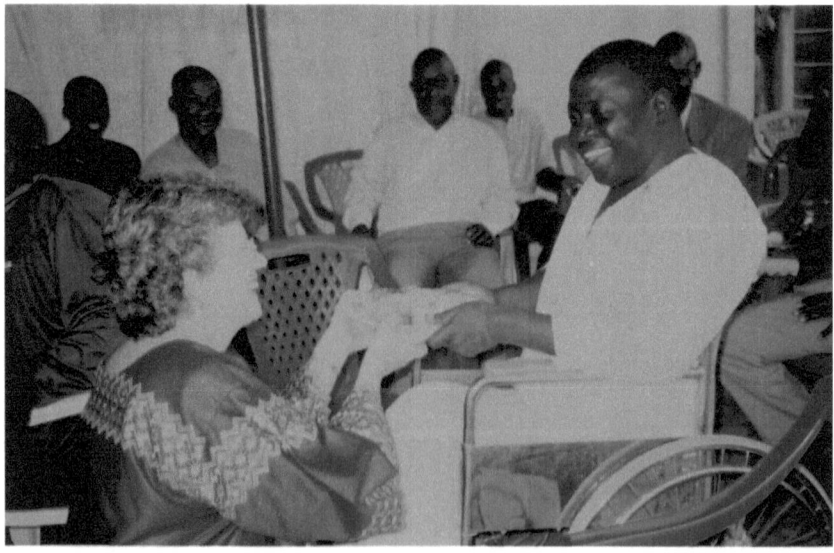

I met Godfrey on a walking clinic. He had been paralysed for 15 years and over time was able to get out of his chair and walk with help. When I knelt, in a Ugandan sign of respect, to serve him lunch at a UACO celebration day, the crowd heaved with emotion.

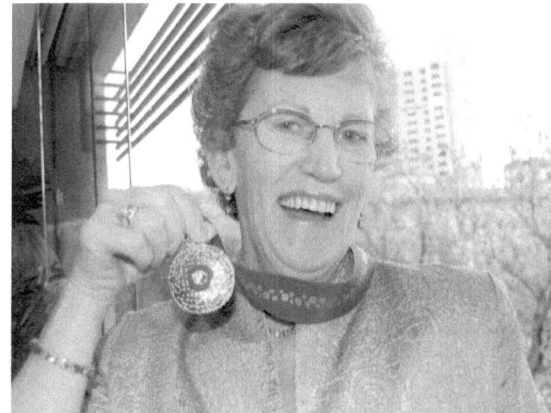

The Order of Australia I received from South Australian Governor Marjorie Jackson-Nelson at Government House, Adelaide 2006.

Wash day Uganda style – me with my twin tub!

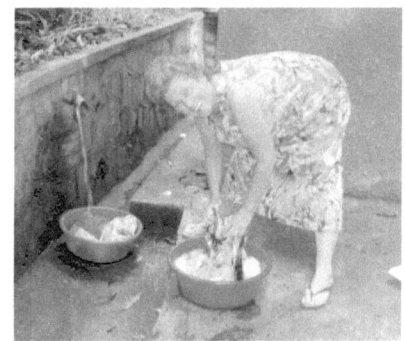

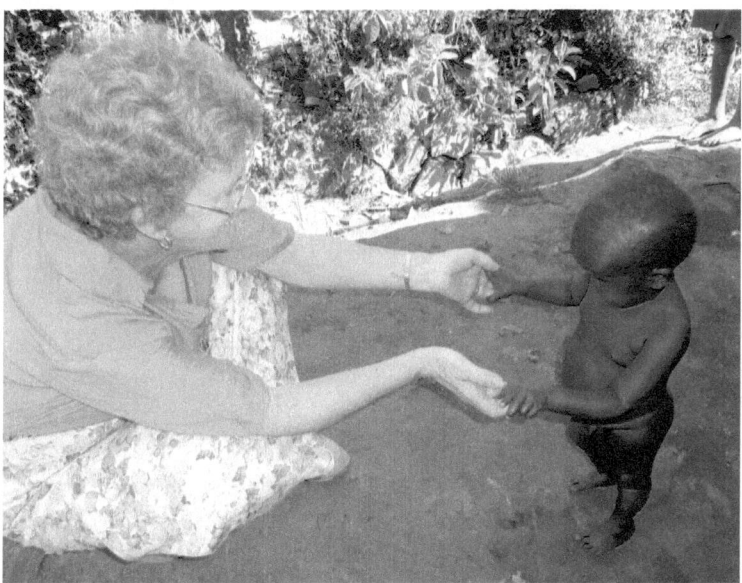

'Walking clinics' through the villages and slums always produced unexpected moments of delight.

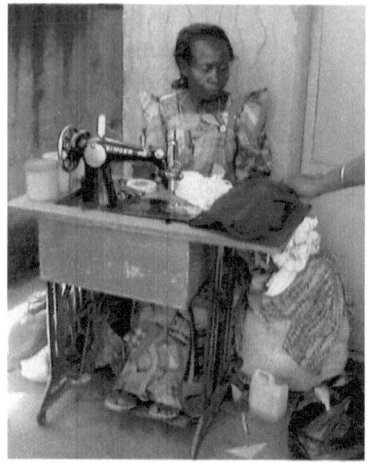

One of the AIDS widows rents a one-metre square section of the clinic verandah, where she runs a sewing business.

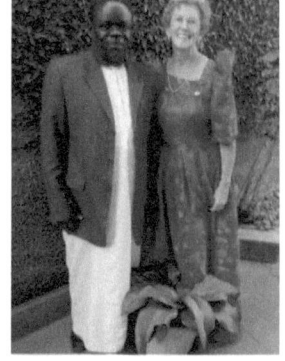

Dr Edward Ssembatya and me – founders of UACO.

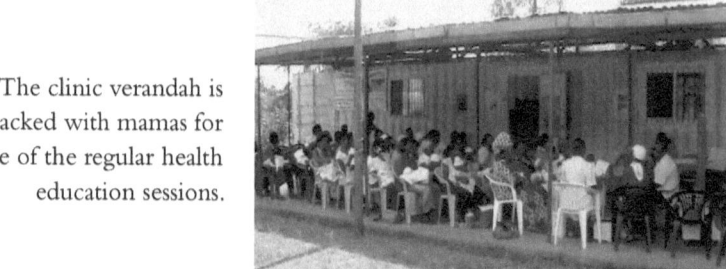

The clinic verandah is packed with mamas for one of the regular health education sessions.

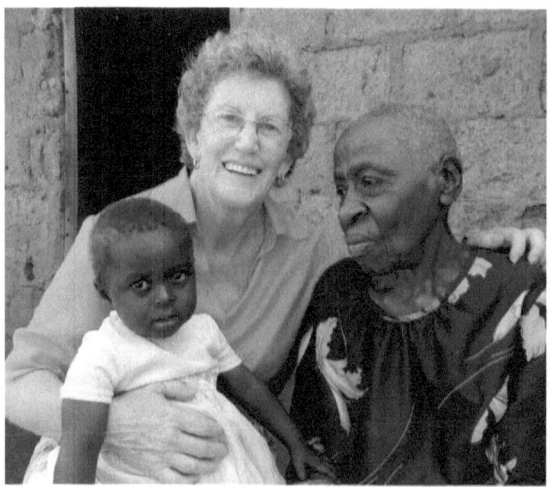

AIDS often leaves the very old having to care for the very young. This young girl has only her great-grandmother to look after her.

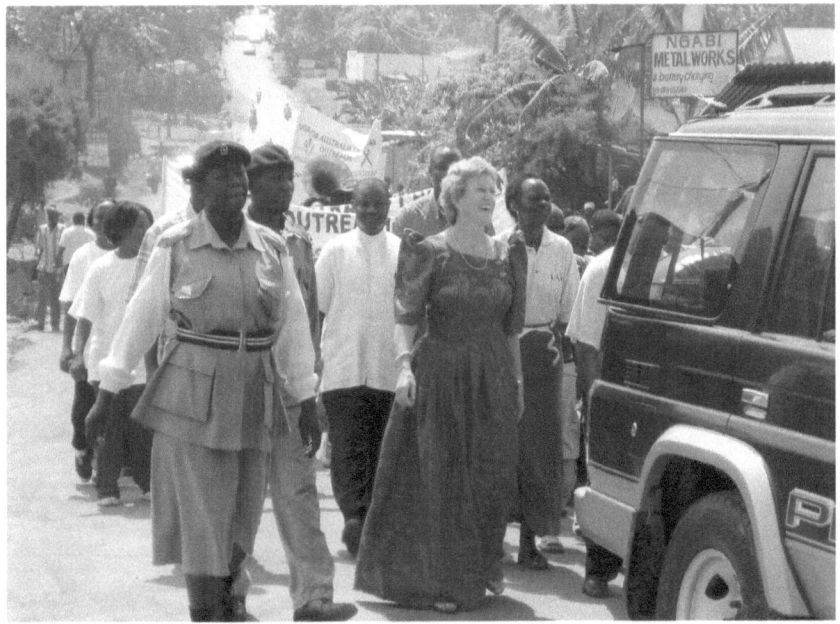

The funding from the Australian Government through AusAID was celebrated with a march through the streets of Kampala to the sounds of a brass band. It delayed the traffic, including the car of the Vice-President.

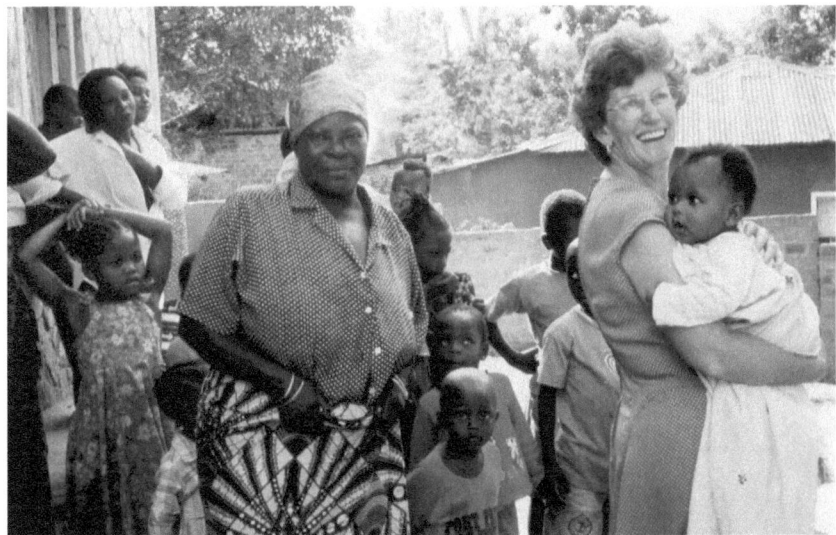

A 'walking clinic' in Nakulabye. These are home visits to the sick and elderly who are unable to come to the clinic for treatment. At first we could only reach those who lived near the clinic, but now the staff go further afield.

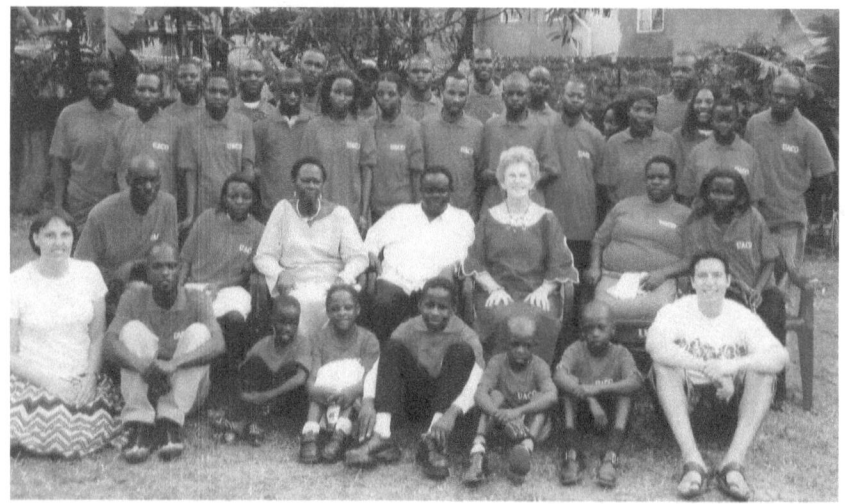

The youth group in 2008 with Iva, Persis, Edward, me and Anthony.

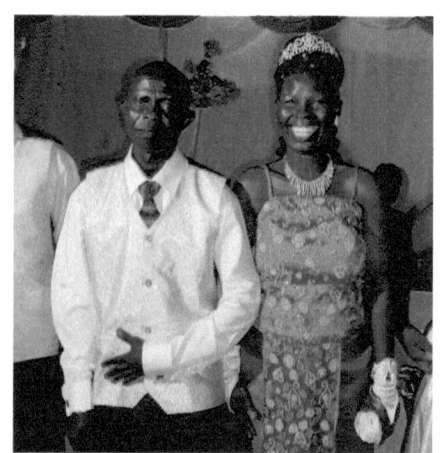

Johnson and Pauline on their wedding day. Although both have AIDS, their marriage was celebrated in true Ugandan style with much dancing.

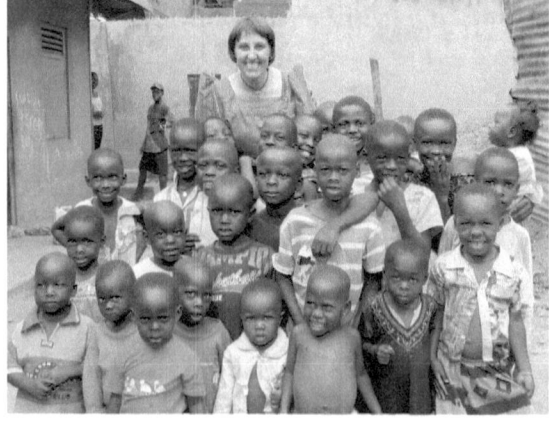

Iva Quarisa has a beautiful heart for people and she is like the Pied Piper when she visits Uganda. My hope is that one day she will take over the running of UACO.

made little difference. Eventually Edward insisted I see a *mzungu* doctor, an Englishman who diagnosed a pinched nerve in my spine. He prescribed some anti-inflammatory pills and stretching exercises. After a few days my aches eased, but I was still undecided about whether to go on the walking clinic or not. Then I thought to myself, I didn't come over here to sit on my butt. We walked for what seemed an eternity that day, up and down in the oppressive heat, and I didn't suffer any ill effects. I found out after my return home that I had developed bursitis, an inflammation of the joint.

One morning Recheal, the nurse from the Florence Nightingale Clinic whose training I was sponsoring, joined me on a walking clinic. I was impressed with her confident and gentle manner. I gave her four text books for her training and some new clothes, and she wrote me a beautiful letter of welcome and thanksgiving, not just for what I was doing for her but for the people of Uganda.

As we walked around the village there were many sick *jajas*, but they were always excited to see us. We went into their homes and sat while these dear old women went around and greeted everyone on their knees. I knew it was the custom but still found it difficult to allow an old woman to do this. On this clinic I also found two toddlers, both aged about two, both suffering as a result of inept injections given to them at a small clinic somewhere in Najjanankumbi. I made a note to speak to Edward about how we could counter this sort of malpractice.

On another walking clinic we found great-grandfather Anthony again. Last time he was caring for six children, but this time he was alone and it was hard to find out what had happened to the children. He was almost blind, with cataracts on both eyes, and so could only move about in his immediate environment. We took him some food, soap and vaseline, and his face lit up. He was so excited and grateful.

One day I met a tiny *jaja* named Noellina who was paralysed from the waist down. She moved by dragging herself along the ground with her hands; her palms looked like the heels of her feet and her knees were badly calloused. She was sitting in the dirt (which was mud, because it had been raining) trying to wash her clothes because she had diarrhoea.

I found a young woman named Prossy nearby who rented a room in Noellina's house, and she said that another woman bathes her on the weekend. I asked Prossy how much rent she paid and said the answer was 5000 shillings per month (A$4.50). I told her she was getting very cheap rent and that it would be a good idea if she took care of the old woman. For this I got a shrug of the shoulders and a response that she gave the old woman one meal a day. I saw the pile of rags on the floor where Noellina slept while someone else slept on the large bed in the same filthy room. By this time my nurse from the hospital was in tears, but I was too angry to cry. I kept on working away at Prossy and she agreed she could take better care of the old woman and that she would bathe her in the middle of the week. I left drugs for Noellina to clear up the diarrhoea.

When I got back to the clinic I called Edward and Florence together for a meeting. Edward immediately caught on to my anger and distress. I told him that this woman was being treated worse than a dog – strong language to use in discussion with a Ugandan. Arrangements were made for three widows to clean her house. The hospital carpenter was commissioned to make her a bed which was close to the ground so she could lift herself into it, and it came with a new mattress and sheets.

In the weeks that followed we had the floor cemented and a ramp built so Noellina could use it to crawl in and out of her house. She asked if there was any money left over to help with the cold wind that comes in the window (a hole with bars on it, covered by a bag and a piece of tin at night); the carpenter installed shutters. I had found that two women lived in this house (Prossy and another one) paying minimal rent so I lined them up and asked them if they liked to have nice bedrooms. When they said yes I told them that our *jaja* also liked and deserved to have a nice room, and that they were to clear the rubbish out of her room and keep it so that she could get in and out of her bed. They understood, particularly when I explained that if they didn't I would clean it out myself and burn the lot when I next visited. They also knew that I had reported them to the head woman of the village and she would be keeping her eye on them.

In the weeks that followed I had a lovely surprise when two women came to thank me for what we were doing for Noellina. One was her daughter and the other the woman who slept in the other bed and apparently looked after her in the evenings. We spoke about her needs and right to receive care, food and love.

Even then in my fourth year in Uganda, there were still plenty of cultural communication breakdowns. One morning, Flavia from the widows group committee came to the office asking me to their meeting (which I knew nothing about). When we started the meeting the chairwoman and one other committee member were missing. I politely told them there would be no meeting unless the chair was there along with all members of the committee, so we then spent some time talking generally about their lives. When I went back to the hospital, Edward was chuckling and said, 'I told them you would not have the meeting unless they were all there.'

Another of the communication frustrations was to make plain that UACO was not about handing out money endlessly. Time and again I would ask for some ideas regarding ways we could support the widows and orphans and the answers would be simply to give more money for medicines, increased salaries or equipment. We needed to find sustainable ways to administer primary health and generate income. If I just had a handout mentality, it would be possible for me to step off the plane every time I came and hand a UACO cheque over and fly home again. We needed schemes to improve life and empower communities in the long term.

I had given handouts particularly in Nakulabye, largely due to the generosity of friends in Australia who had given money for me to use where needed. But we had learnt lessons along the way. The UACO committee in Australia, in consultation with Edward, had decided we wanted to develop an emphasis on empowerment rather than paternalism.

Other breakdowns had nothing to do with Africans but African infrastructure. One day I went to Edward's office to use the computer while he was out. I tried ringing Edward but the phones weren't working. After a while they came good so I spoke to him, but during that time the power went off. When it returned the computer seized up and had to be switched on and off, losing the morning's work. Even sending an email home could be a drama and I had regular and frustrating conversations with technical people trying to find a better way. Mostly it was to no avail, so when I found a connection that was online and working I would tend to send everything I could, fearing it would crash any second.

In contrast to the e-frustrations, I was thrilled with the way things were being run. Florence and Edward both understood my obsession with transparency. They kept good records and Edward showed again that his generosity extended beyond his medical care for others. The bank account we opened for UACO last year didn't come through for three months but this didn't stop bills mounting up for the clinic, so Edward personally paid them. Even when 17 million shillings (then about A$15,000) from the Canadian consulate was deposited in the account to pay for the cows, he didn't touch it until I had looked through the books. He was happy to be reimbursed when I was satisfied all was in order. Edward, to use his own words, understands money.

It still took many, many hours to go through all the receipts and notes and match everything up. I found it exhausting and, despite reciting 'TIA' over and over in my head, eventually I needed to act. Help came in the form of Bukenya, who administered and handled the accounts at Edward's hospital. He agreed to help manage the UACO accounts and the small loan scheme, which was a tremendous relief. I was realising that my role was changing within UACO toward administration rather than nursing – although the two positions would remain intricately woven.

Chapter Sixteen

THE LOCAL PAPERS WERE full of the rumblings of tribal politics. Celebrations including a military parade were to be staged in honour of the downfall of Idi Amin – some twenty-three years after the event. According to President Museveni's political secretary, Moses Byaruhanga, the cabinet decided the overthrow of the former dictator hadn't been given the necessary attention in the past. The idea was that a celebration of his downfall would now be an annual event to encourage unity and stability. Apparently the cabinet had agreed on the celebration last year but hadn't managed to organise it until now in April 2002. There was talk about Obote being allowed back to live in Uganda, but Edward said that would never happen while Museveni was in power – that is, unless there was another civil war.

I was getting desperate for a break or, more specifically, some sleep – the hostel was as noisy as ever, with much late-night partying. Rather than escaping again to the Sheraton, this time I booked a short holiday at a Nile River resort at Jinja, north-east of Kampala.

The weekend didn't get off to a great start when it rained heavily the night before and the road to Jinja became a bog. I grew worried when the driver started slowing, because in Uganda there is only one speed – flat out. We groaned and creaked our way to the resort signpost and proceeded down a very muddy road. Eventually the driver said he couldn't go any further and that it was 'just round the corner'. I got out of the car and walked in the mud, slipping, sliding and praying all the time. I finally made it to the resort, leaving my mud-caked shoes at the front entrance. It took another five hours before my room was available, a little cottage consisting of a bedroom and lounge with a TV that only showed a 24-hour sports channel. I didn't really care because I had a book to read and from the little balcony I could watch the Nile. Men were fishing from small boats and on the other bank women were doing their washing. There were some rapids here and there, and sometimes you could see tourists canoeing down them. Mostly I slept or rested, which was the point of the whole exercise.

I returned feeling refreshed and decided it was time to pay Frank and Michele a visit. Their circumstances had changed. They had moved from the house I shared with them on my first journey to Uganda and were now living in terrible conditions. In some parts of the house there were no ceilings, fly screens or inside plumbing. There were even rats and mice, although they had a cat to act as a deterrent. They had built their own church and started a small school in Lugala, a slum area on the western part of Kampala. It was about a forty-five minute drive from the Busabala Road clinic and occasionally they would bring sick or dying people there for free treatment. Other than that we met socially a few times when I was in Uganda to share our experiences and senses of humour.

Michele and I visited Suzan, the orphan sponsored by my daughter, who was at a boarding school. She was eight years old now and looked gorgeous and grabbed me into a huge hug. I gave her a recent photo of Fiona and she put it with her precious things. She had grown taller and a teacher told us she was very bright and well liked. Michele gave her a large bag of sweets which Suzan, without prompting, took outside and shared with all of the other children. Her medical condition continued to be precarious, however, because her keloid scarring was again preventing her from standing properly as she grew. I took Suzan to see Edward and he believed that soon she would need more extensive surgery.

When I returned to UACO, the youth group's first football match was a scene of much excitement. The directors of UACO (that is, Edward and me) were officially introduced to both teams. Our boys looked very smart in their new t-shirts with the UACO logo on them, though the footwear wasn't so consistent. Some played barefoot, some had sneakers while others wore odd, very worn-out boots. The pitch was dirt with fine, loose stones sprayed across it, the potholes filled with soil-stuffed plastic bags. UACO won four-nil, with great screams of delight accompanying every goal (particularly from me).

We shouted them all a soft drink afterwards and, as usual, I had to make a speech, which I used to tell our boys how excited and proud we were of them. After some photos I taught them to chant 'UACO! UACO! Go! Go! Go!', which caused more laughter, and now everyone in Najjanankumbi knew about the *mzungu* who goes to the football.

Soon after, Edward spent a week in Tripoli at an AIDS conference and the timing couldn't have been worse as the hospital was overrun with patients. As torrential rain bucketed down, we were run off our feet in the clinic due to some very sick babies with malaria, probably as a result of the rain.

While Edward was away, standards and effort quickly started slipping at the hospital. A radio blared on the nurses' desk while a very sick person was in a bed next door. The driver and car disappeared without telling anyone and we needed to send a patient to Mulago urgently. And despite always being instructed to light the furnace in the evening, the cleaners lit it during the day and filled the clinic with choking grey smoke.

A few hospital staff members were shocked when I came through the corridors and gave them some lessons in how things should be done. Playing the parts of auditor, director of nursing and general dragon lady, I pulled my weight all over the hospital, reprimanding staff for being lazy, sleeping on duty and ignoring their patients and equipment. I even shouted at one snoozing cleaner and threatened to sack him; he was not happy. When I stopped for lunch with Rose, she was delighted and laughed when I told her that the word was out: 'Don't mess with *mzungu* mama!' In a short time the hospital was pulled into shape again.

It turned out Edward's week at the AIDS 'conference' was a giant scam by Gaddafi. He had brought together, at his own cost, 600 ministers and doctors from all over the continent to explain how he wanted to be president of a United States of Africa. They were taken from Tripoli to his palace at Benghazi where he and his ministers spoke about the need for African unity. The only mention of AIDS was that there is 'a problem', an unnecessary understatement to say the least. Gaddafi finished with a tirade against the USA and Israel, and Edward returned with a head cold but without his baggage.

I can barely describe how wonderful the day was when Allan arrived. The days leading up to it were spent cleaning the tiny room at the hostel and trying to overcome a bout of illness; I had some symptoms of malaria but a test proved negative. I was so ill one weekend I could barely get out of bed, so I spent much time imagining where Allan would be on the flight and what he was doing.

I met him at Entebbe airport and, after lunch with Edward and Rose, we unpacked at the hostel. In no time Allan had the cork out of a bottle of Penfolds red which we drank accompanied by an African fruit salad and a beautiful sunset. We had so much to catch up on and just talked and talked and talked. The long and winding conversation included a discussion about the future of UACO, and I concluded that this would be my last time working in Uganda. I was now almost sixty, I had regular aches and pains to contend with, the travel costs were expensive and I missed Allan too much. We agreed to rethink our commitment to UACO because we felt it was time for others to be involved and take over some roles. I felt firm in my resolve, but in the back of my mind I was aware that I had been so in the past – would God have other plans for me?

Allan's first day at work was an experience for everyone. The minute I got there Edward whisked Allan off to show him around while I was still downloading my email in the office, and I suddenly realised he had taken Allan out to the clinic and was introducing him to everyone. I was furious, not to mention incredibly hurt that he had not included me. I told Edward that I didn't mind him showing Allan around the hospital, but the clinic was my heart's work. Edward has never seen me so cross. I understood his excitement but I was hurt. He was very sorry and apologised profusely.

Allan was given a formal welcome at the clinic by both the widows and the youths. We both made speeches, during which we told them we would buy the youth group some African drums to replace the plastic jerry cans they had been using.

After observing the mayhem of the clinic, the following day Allan had his first look at the life of the people of Najjanankumbi. As we walked the locals called out to me as usual using various names, while Allan looked like the Pied Piper with about twenty kids running behind him at one stage. The noise was incredible;

I wondered if they had ever seen a white man there before. My *jajas* were so pleased to meet him. It was important for me too that Allan saw how hard the work was, how great the humanity, and the reasons I was so worn out and yet enamored of Africa.

He later told me how struck he was by the poverty of the people the clinic reached. There was no government health care, unemployment benefits or pensions here. People sleep on bags, cardboard or papers on a dirt floor; most do not have water, electricity or sewerage. Amid this he also saw the hope and joy people felt when they received the benefits of what the clinic provided. In addition to being able to show Uganda to Allan, it was wonderful to discuss the administrative stuff with him. He helped write the final budget which we explained in detail during meetings with Edward, Rose, Florence and Bukenya. They were all pleased and agreed that UACO should concentrate on free medical outreach for the needy.

In between work we slipped away to see the source of the Nile River and the beautiful Bujaghali Falls at Jinja. In Kampala we visited a craft market and saw ebony being carved, had a cold beer at the Sheraton and caught a *boda-boda* up the hill to All Saints Church. The service was louder and more Pentecostal than Allan was used to but he enjoyed the sermon. For me it is Africa; there is nothing quite as wonderful as resonant African voices raised in song and I always love it. The men in particular singing 'Amazing Grace' is something I will never forget.

Edward asked if we wanted to visit the equator zone, which is about an hour's drive south-east of Kampala. As we headed off Allan started feeling poorly, which I at first put down to some travel sickness combined with the diesel fumes. By the time we returned to the compound it had progressed from stomach aches to the point where he couldn't walk and was white as a sheet. He lay on the floor of Edward's office looking like a cadaver.

We put him into one of the hospital beds and as we treated him I saw a suitcase near the end of his bed with sheets from Australia in it. The writing on the case was Allan's. He had gone full circle: having packed the bed and mattress he was now using them on the other side of the world. Rose brought him black African tea with ginger in it. Allan eventually got down two cups and I got him dressed and home to the hostel to recover.

It took several days for Allan to get back on his feet, so he was unable to visit Recheal at the hospital at Kiwoko with me, a one and a half hour drive to the north toward Sudan. Recheal was so excited to see me and the gifts I had brought. I met the hospital's medical superintendent to get an update on how she was going and to pay her fees for the next twelve months, plus some extra for clothes, text books and stationery. It added up to about $2000, which I paid for.

In the final days before Allan and I were due to fly out, we transferred the money from UACO Australia into the bank account in Kampala to fulfill the UACO budget and began a series of farewells, starting with the *jajas* on our walking clinic through the village. Allan and I bought groceries for Anna-Mary and Beth. They were living in the most deplorable conditions, but Beth was well and happy enough. We gave Beth some books and crayons and she read to us. She had improved much since last year. Anna-Mary had prepared lunch and soon started on about what she wanted, but I had become adept at setting boundaries regarding what I could and couldn't provide. We left enough money with Frank and Michele to pay three months rent in advance when she found a bigger room.

We then visited Alice at the Florence Nightingale Clinic in Nakulabye. She was expecting us and so was in her best dress and high-heeled shoes. There was a brand new baby boy there and Allan was asked to name him. He suggested Joshua, explaining to the mother that Joshua had saved many people's lives and was a good man. Thomas was there as usual but he looked so thin. Allan handed out some sweets and it caused a stampede; one little tot who could not have been more than two came tearing across the compound in full voice and pushed her way to the front.

After the mayhem died down, we went with Alice and a nurse to visit three AIDS patients. This way Allan was able to see the slums of Nakulabye without raising too many suspicions. The people still remembered me there, otherwise they would have been very suspicious about a couple of *mzungus* walking about their village. I have always thought it an intrusion to go into the slums where I am unknown and so take things gently until they understand why I am there. I think it is fair to say that Allan had his eyes opened.

Our final farewell was to Florence, Edward and Rose. Their faces hit the floor when I told them I wouldn't be back next year and I had tears in my eyes too. I explained that the cost of my plane fares, board, food and transport each year came from our savings and that UACO needed to start working towards becoming an African health program, not an Australian handout. I said I thought others might be coming and that I would return in two years time for a shorter visit, but eventually I would not be able to continue making the journey. I promised that I would stay in touch and keenly watch everything that happened, but there needed to be scrupulous Ugandan administration.

Chapter Seventeen

ALLAN HAD FULLY RECOVERED by the time we flew to London to meet his brother, John, and sister-in-law, Rosemary. After a few days catching up with family, the four of us flew to Madeira for a fortnight of Portuguese culture and food.

We came home via Kuala Lumpur to visit Peter and Katrina and our grandsons Michael and Joshua. Peter had been in Malaysia for a year with the army, and their allocated apartment was near to the Petronas Twin Towers in the city. After a lovely family time together, we flew home via Singapore, only to be offloaded there as the aircraft was overbooked. I was told this happens a lot and we were well looked after, including being upgraded to business class for the flight home the next day.

When we arrived home in June 2002 we found the caravan we had ordered earlier in the year was ready. We had had a wonderful time in our off-road camper trailer staying at remote bush camps, but I had no desire to get bogged and marooned again. We decided to buy a small caravan with more creature comforts which would allow us to keep travelling but with less hassles. We planned to visit the boys in Sydney and Brisbane but our maiden journey would be to the Great Australian Bight with Ailee and Fred Wilson, our close church and UACO friends. I had a yearning to see the southern right whales that come from Antarctica to breed in the warmer waters off South Australia during the winter. The contrast of the sheer cliffs of the Nullarbor Plain leading to the sparkling Southern Ocean was stunning. We marvelled at the huge and gentle creatures.

Although I wouldn't be returning to Uganda in 2002, late in that year UACO Australian secretary, Ian Attenborough, went. The visit was deeply moving for him and answered a nagging question he had had for many years. A microbiologist who worked at the Adelaide Children's Hospital for thirty-two years, the seed of caring had been sown in Ian during the late 1960s when he heard a doctor named Ward Derrington speak to a Methodist Youth Fellowship about his experiences working in a hospital in Lahore, Pakistan. Ian had felt the pull to volunteer overseas ever since but never found the opportunity. When he retired in 1997 he wondered if he had misunderstood a call from God, and after working for UACO he decided now was the time. Ian flew to Uganda for ten weeks to offer his skills to Edward's staff in the hospital's small laboratory.

The youth group welcomed him with traditional drums and singing. In addition to playing soccer and volleyball, they had also been involved in community work such as cleaning the village wells, and their first cabbage crop was about to be harvested. The money raised went back into financing youth activities, including planting their next crop, maize. The project brought the group together as they had to prepare the soil, water and weed the crop and protect it from thieves at the time of harvest. Ian was inspired by these young people taking control of their lives, just as I had been.

He also witnessed the suffering of the Congolese refugees, sleeping on mattresses with twelve to twenty to a room, and now about 150 of them in two houses. There was also the warmth of appreciation, including one dignified woman of high standing who sang beautifully in thanks for the food and baby clothes that had been distributed. Ian returned with many photos – a favourite of mine was one of Bosco standing unaided in front of his wheelchair on a walking clinic.

Ian was also in Africa for a significant event when the Nigel Ambler Memorial Conference Room was formally opened. The money donated in lieu of flowers at the memorial service for Gillies' son had been used to furnish and equip the hospital training room. After some speeches, Ian presented an overhead projector to Edward. Although overhead projectors are being phased out in favour of computer projection in Australia, they are hard to come by in Uganda and it was received as a treasured teaching aid. A framed photograph of Nigel and Gillies was placed on the wall.

When Ian returned to Adelaide, it was wonderful hearing first-hand how everyone was going. It seemed the walking and health clinics were busy while the education side was growing. A day had been set aside for young women, and thirty-two teenagers came along for counselling and education on HIV/AIDS. The impact of UACO's work grew with a seminar held where 250 community leaders, such as MPs, government officers, village leaders and police discussed security, crime prevention and community cooperation. Hearing all the news reinforced the fact that, for the past four years, I had spent part of each year preparing to go to Africa, and it felt strange not to be packing my suitcase.

In Australia, I had a formal function to attend on behalf of UACO. Along with Allan, Gillies and Wendy Ambler, I went to Government House in Adelaide because I was a finalist in the Senior Australian of the Year awards. I don't know who nominated me, although I suspect it was someone from Westbourne Park Uniting Church. At first I was absolutely shocked by the nomination, but then felt honoured – I wished everyone involved with UACO could have been honoured in a similar way. It was wonderful recognition for the many people involved in achieving so much for the people of Uganda. The breakfast function was hosted by Bruno Krumins, the Lieutenant Governor of South Australia. The eventual winner was Dr Marie O'Neill for her work as chief psychologist for the South Australian Department of Community Welfare.

In the new year of 2003 we were flying again, this time because our daughter, Fiona, had fallen in love with Warrick Taylor, a delightful Englishman. The wedding was held in a private hotel overlooking Lake Windemere in the beautiful Lake District of England. The ceremony was exquisite; Fiona had decorated the room with dozens of white roses and she looked as simple and elegant as something out of a *Vogue* magazine. Drinks were served on the terrace as guests watched the boats on the lake before a mid afternoon meal. After an early evening rest, a black tie party commenced and went until late. My only regret is that our sons could not join us: Peter was serving in East Timor while David was unable to get time off from Qantas. I really missed them and shed a few tears for Fiona not being able to share this day with her brothers.

The wedding coincided with my sixtieth birthday, and Fiona told everyone except me about a surprise she had planned. Just two weeks after the wedding, we left our husbands in England and Fiona took me to New York for four magnificent days, a place I had often fantasised about. New York was totally captivating. We window-shopped at Tiffany's, rode around Central Park in a horse and carriage and went to the top of the Empire State Building. I told Allan that if I found Cary Grant there (circa *An Affair to Remember*) then I wouldn't be coming back.

Back in Australia, UACO was never far from my mind and even began changing our caravanning schedule as our itinerary was manipulated to fit in speaking to groups along the way. Our final destinations were Sydney and Brisbane to see the boys and their families but Mount Gambier was first on the list, and it was wonderful for Mum to come and listen for the first time to what her daughter had been up to. She had certainly been challenged by the changes in my life and at first it cannot have been easy for her. As a Catholic, she found it difficult to accept I would give up Catholicism to join the Uniting Church, then give up a very good job to go to Africa. But afterwards she told me she was very proud of the work I was doing, and for me that was wonderful.

We used the trip to head over the border into southern New South Wales, and finally take up Luigi and Mary Quarisa's offer of a cuppa in Griffith, the couple who had so generously donated to the project after seeing it on *The 7.30 Report*. As soon as we drove onto their farm we felt at home, and the cuppa turned into an overnight stay at 'Hotel Quarisa' – the first of many happy visits. Luigi peppered me with questions about UACO and our conversations then spread into deep discussions about the world.

We met the rest of the family and it was clear Luigi and Mary had raised their family to have generous hearts. One of their daughters, Iva, showed a particular interest in Uganda. She had a science degree and was working with the New South Wales government as a natural resource management adviser. Iva later began financially supporting UACO and made inquiries about travelling to Uganda with me.

We also met up with Julie Lomax in Redhead, on the coast near Newcastle, to thank her and her band of willing helpers for their work and generosity. She sent us on our way with two more large bags of toys.

As well as meeting UACO supporters, these trips gave me a chance to speak to many others about the project. I was, and continue to be, amazed at the breadth and diversity of people and organisations who give financially, prayerfully or in kind.

I spoke to large groups at Penrith, Port Macquarie and Alstonville in New South Wales and was touched that some people travelled long distances to hear about UACO. When I spoke of the plight of the poor and marginalised in Uganda, I didn't hold back. I used slides to tell the stories of malaria, HIV/AIDS, poverty and malnutrition, showing the faces of Uganda.

After one talk, a man approached me about ongoing funding. He was an academic who, with the help of another man, ran a book and gift shop to raise funds for charity. They had been supporting a project that had come to an end and were interested in UACO. After discussions with Fred Wilson, they generously offered $1000 to start a micro-loan scheme for widows and youth for income-generating projects. They would continue that level of funding for the next two years until their shop lease came to an end. Up until now, we had only taken tiny steps towards setting up a loan scheme, and the widows had offered to contribute 200 shillings (15 cents) each at every meeting to build up a fund. Edward, in his wisdom, had already set up a small loans management committee, although at the time he had no prospect of funding. His committee had already established strict guidelines for repayment and interest rates and so was ready to begin with this new source of funds.

With the finances now available, Bukenya conducted training days on how to handle the loans and make an application. Soon sixteen widows were approved for loans ranging between $40 and $150. They planned to develop a range of small businesses. With the piggeries, market gardens and now a true micro-loan scheme, UACO was finally also having an economic impact on the people of Najjanankumbi rather than just giving medical help.

The micro-loan scheme soon raised another area of need. Most adults couldn't apply for a loan because they couldn't read or write. Many would not even be able to sign their name at the bottom of an application form, let alone fill it in. Anthony Radford stresses the link between illiteracy and poverty and quotes a study in forty-five countries that showed that a one per cent increase in women's literacy was three times more likely to improve the health of women and children than a one per cent increase in the number of doctors. Edward's executive committee asked if we would support an adult literacy group. UACO had money in the bank in Australia from various donations and we immediately paid to get a classroom started. It would cost about $30 per month to hire a teacher. The classroom was in the Nigel Ambler conference room on the top floor of the hospital.

In August 2003, the youth group and the widows submitted a proposal to raise pigs and they believed it would make them self-sufficient. Their plan included several sites, buying, feeding and breeding pigs, and earning a profit from the sale of fattened pigs. If successful, it not only offered the chance to provide an income for mostly unemployed people, but it would also boost their self-esteem. The UACO committee was so impressed with the submission that we agreed to assist with the initial cost of establishing the piggery. We wrote to Australians who had donated to UACO in the past, asking if they would sponsor a pig at a cost of $20. The response was wonderful, and by the end of the year $2500 had been raised to help buy more than 100 piglets and pay some veterinary fees. Training days were held to teach those involved about treating mange, worms and iron deficiency. Shortly after this, I received an email from the leader of the youth group, Ronny Mutebi, entitled 'It's a new day'.

> *Indeed it's a new day, new hope for a brighter future. On 23 August 2003 we received the first batch of pigs. It was such an excitement as everyone got involved in the offloading of the piglets, preparing the feeds. Oh God, words can't express it all.*
>
> *This project is not only an income-generating activity but also a time occupant for the youth. The youth have acquired skills in pig husbandry at the centre.*
>
> *There has been a change in youths' behaviour and I would like to take this opportunity to thank you so much for your generosity and changing the lives of many youth who thought [they] could never make anything out of their lives. Not forgetting Dr Ssembatya, we thank you so much for being father to the fatherless and opening your home to us. May the Almighty bless you all and reward you abundantly.*

About the same time, Edward wrote that the physiotherapy department had opened at his hospital with equipment that had all been donated from Australia and sent in the container. He gave an example of how it had already been used. A 58-year-old widow from the UACO group had had a stroke four years before and came to the clinic weak, lacking co-ordination and depressed. She was so debilitated that she couldn't manage steps or access the toilet. Her rehabilitation gave her new strength, increased mobility and less pain.

After almost two years away from Uganda I was anticipating a return in 2004. However, in January I received a phone call to say Mum had been suddenly admitted to hospital in Mount Gambier. After three days of investigations, the doctors advised us the prognosis was not good and Allan and I left immediately to be with her. She died surrounded by us all, fully cognisant that she was dying and truly peaceful.

Chapter Eighteen

Despite my yearning to return to Uganda, to be honest, the reality of being back there felt harder than any other year. It was May 2004. The heat and dust seemed to affect me more, but it didn't help that I arrived already tired. The months leading up to this trip had been spent dealing with Mum's death. Peter and Katrina's family increased with the birth of their third son, Timothy Andrew, in March, and we had also been anticipating the birth of Fiona and Warrick's first child. Allan flew to the UK to help Warrick with house renovations, then I flew in a month later in time for the arrival of John Laurence Taylor. While Allan had to return to Australia soon after little John's birth, I stayed to help out for a couple of weeks before flying on to Uganda.

Edward had worked out a packed six-week program for me, during which Florence would show me everything that had been going on since my last visit. Edward didn't want to discuss the budget until I had the full inspection, because much had changed in two years. I avoided the hostel this time around and stayed at Michele and Frank Heyward's house. They had now been in Uganda for five years and had moved out of the dilapidated house they had been in and were now in a comfortable house in Lugala, the low-lying slum area in Kampala, where they had built a church and school last time I was there. It was wonderful to stay with old friends and talk about life there and at home, plus I had room to move around and was free to make my own meals. The Heywards also had a lovely twenty-nine-year-old house girl named Pauline, who was well advanced with AIDS but able to cope with the work.

It took only one drive to bring back the memory of clogged roads and potholes. Edward lent me his car and driver and after heavy rain, the forty-five-minute drive into the clinic was now a boggy mess. I later suggested to Allan via email that we spend the $1000 it would take to concrete the road from the gate right up to the hospital door as a matter of urgency.

Despite the muddy entrance, it was so exciting to see the clinic again. Some of the plants that the goats 'pruned' two years ago had grown back, and two trees were growing well. They had planted mulinga trees, which are highly valued in Uganda as the leaves are high in vitamins and minerals so are used as a vegetable. Often the leaves are dried and used to make tea by HIV/AIDS patients, while oil from the seed is used as a cream on the body. But the medicinal parts are the stems and roots, which are crushed into powder and mixed with water before being drunk. They are said to cure many diseases by helping the body's metabolism.

It was immunisation day and it was thrilling to see people coming. In addition to the mamas and babies, there were about fifty people waiting for treatment. Initially patients are seen by the nurse, Ronald Kayiwa, and if he cannot manage the problem in the clinic then they are sent over to the hospital to see Edward. Walking around, I was amused to see an enormous framed photo of Edward with Allan and me from my last trip taking pride of place in Edward's office. Fiona's wedding photo was pinned to his noticeboard and another inside the clinic.

The clinic was now open two days per week for medical services and immunisations; the other days it was used for counselling and meetings. On the walking clinics, widows were always looking for mothers and babies they didn't recognise or who needed immunisation explained to them. There were fewer pregnant women in Najjanankumbi, proof that family planning education was paying off. I was so excited to see the plans being fulfilled. When I thought back to when the clinic first started and so few mothers understood anything about family planning, some serious inroads were now being made.

The expansion of clinic services included the work of a physiotherapist, Lubega, who volunteered one day per week. Edward didn't have the money to pay him and there were only a few patients. He was a lovely young man who passionately wanted to do his Master of Rehabilitation; there are only three people with this qualification in all of Uganda but the course cost about $1000 per year. Lubega had asked Edward if he could set up a rehabilitation clinic in what used to be his original house next to the hospital, as Edward had now moved. Lubega said there were many people he could help such as those who had suffered strokes, arthritis, sporting or car accidents, if he had more equipment. He needed hand, arm and leg braces and adjustable parallel bars so both adults and children could use them.

One of Lubega's patients was forty-five years old and had suffered a stroke. She was paralysed on the left side and couldn't talk. After undergoing treatment, she started walking using a stick; her left arm was in a sling and couldn't be rehabilitated but she could talk slowly. In some ways, rehabilitation is the least glamorous work, but so many people in Uganda are completely and unnecessarily housebound and need help.

Edward and Florence presented me with a huge number of folders to audit. Looking through them, it was clear that everything in the past two years had been noted. The loan scheme documentation was particularly remarkable: it had been operating for two months without any problems and all twenty-four people involved had repaid on time. There was a well-constructed process of application, recommendation, interview and then loan. As I audited, every single piece of paper or docket was in the correct place. It was simply outstanding.

It was exciting to see the micro-loan scheme in action. The pigs looked great and were well cared for. One of the widows spent so much time with her sow that it became the family pet

– as soon as she scratched the pig's ears it would lay down for more. The youth group had several pens with two boars and seven sows, two of which were expecting a litter. Everyone was very excited about their ventures and it was thrilling to see the loans helping those involved both financially and in building self-esteem.

A friend from the hostel, Julie Bolz, got in contact to say she was returning home to America. Before she flew out, we toured the hospital and clinic together; she was amazed and suggested contacting Bill Gates for support. We had previously applied to the Bill Gates Foundation but were told the only money available was for AIDS research. It did make me think about what could be achieved if we managed to raise the money for the operating theatre or an extension of services for AIDS sufferers, especially by offering the expensive and life-enhancing drugs that we just couldn't afford. That night I was surprised when Allan emailed suggesting perhaps the need for another container.

It all came against a horrible backdrop of lost medical services in Uganda. Edward was desperate to expand the hospital to include a theatre, delivery room, recovery area and consulting rooms, because Mulago Hospital was in a dreadful mess. Mulago is the size of a major public hospital in Australia and was about eight kilometers from Busabala Road. The doctors had recently been on strike because they lacked basic resources such as gloves (let alone drugs), and some of the time they weren't even being paid.

As a result, women in labour had died because they needed Caesarean sections. Accident victims and other patients died while lined up in the corridors, waiting to see doctors. People were told to go home because hospital staff could do nothing for them. And there was talk of further strike action.

Several doctors asked Edward if they could work with him at Busabala Road Hospital – all they needed was a theatre suite. These were senior consultants, including an obstetrician/gynecologist and an orthopedic surgeon. There was a lot to think about. If we brought out another container then perhaps it should focus on setting up the operating theatre; we already had the table and anaesthetic machine. Allan, Fred and Ailee all emailed how excited they were about the possibility of another container and the expansion of the clinic. It seemed as though our home was about to become a warehouse again, with Allan and Fred already collecting equipment from various places. Edward was so excited he couldn't sleep thinking about it all.

Despite the hot and dusty conditions, my first walking clinic was full of laughter, tears and prayers as we handed out beans, sugar and soap. When I spoke to one of the *jajas* in Luganda, she did a double take and asked how I knew her language. The others told her my name here is *Nambatya*, a term applied to some women meaning 'you do not have enemies, everything is handled by God' (the same meaning that Edward's surname, *Ssembatya*, has for men).

The stifling humidity at the tail end of the wet season in May was taking its toll on me on walking clinics, but it wasn't my only concern. I had a flare up of my arthritis and the injections I'd had after a similar event back in Adelaide seemed to have had little effect. My bones ached, with one finger on my left hand and my right thumb ceasing to work for several days. It did ease after some medication.

I was feeling quite off when I went to a meeting of the Kisakye widows at Masajja, the slum area next to Najjanankumbi. Masajja was now included in the walking clinics and so some widows from that area were involved with UACO projects. There were about thirty widows there, all in their best dresses. After some wonderful speeches of welcome came discussions about the loan scheme and pigs. Then the fun started. They sang and danced and even got me up to dance, teaching me to get my rear end going the Ugandan way, all the time screaming with delight. Then I was presented with three lovely baskets with my name woven into them, three pineapples, two hands of bananas, a two-metre long stick of sugar cane and probably three dozen avocados. I went feeling less than well but returned feeling totally blessed.

I took some of these Masajja widows with me on a piggery tour a few days later. For three hours we wandered up and down the hills, over piles of rubbish, through *matoke* (plantain) groves until we were smothered in the fine red dust of the Busabala Road. The pigs were, with only one exception, in very good condition.

Things got a bit silly when I was asked to name them all: I started out with Wilbur and Hermione, which were names sent to us in response to our call for donations to buy pigs. Then I resorted to Matilda and Babe and got stuck, so suggested Judy. This turned out to the name they had all been waiting for, and then anticipation began building about who would have the honour of naming one of their boars Allan. Eventually I ran out of names so resorted to the Bible: Rachel, Rebecca, Esther and Sarah. We decided they were all strong women and so these pigs should grow up to be equally strong and deliver strong babies. The last pig was very cheeky, resting her two front legs over the pen and almost smiling. Raising pigs seemed the way to go in this area because there was a ready demand for pork by the butchers selling from roadside stalls.

Although there was little we could do to treat those with AIDS, we decided to start an AIDS support group at the clinic. This was a challenge because the disease carries such a stigma that many people refuse to even acknowledge they are sick. There were twenty women (and no men) at the first meeting, and I told them how proud I was to see them there. It takes courage to make such a public statement about their illness, and their bravery saw the group grow as more women sought help. Edward gave an excellent blackboard lecture on what we could and could not do for them. One of the victims was sleeping at her father's house, and they had forgotten to lock the door when a man broke in, raped and infected her. She was nine years old at the time; it was all I could do not to cry. She looked really ill and I suspected she wouldn't live for many more years – maybe not even one more. I just wanted to put my arms around her. She was eighteen years old but looked much older.

In contrast, most of the babies brought to the clinic by their mamas were in great shape. They were gorgeous and chubby and captured my heart. It was easy to spot those who were struggling when they arrived for immunisations, so we would steer them to the nurse, Ronald, for extra attention. One day a baby boy of about six months old, wearing a pair of pants fashioned out of some men's trousers, was crying. I picked him up and he stopped and stared at my white face with the biggest brown eyes, then gurgled and smiled. Later, as the clinic was nearing an end, I was sitting inside waiting for the nurse to finish when a little boy about three years old crawled up onto my lap. He snuggled in, chattering away in Luganda, then said goodbye and went home after his mama had seen the nurse. In those moments I felt blessed: I had been homesick and tired and suddenly felt loved and needed.

In between regular commitments at the clinic, it was wonderful to see the progress many old friends were making. Little Thomas, who I had met as a scruffy, scarred, three-year-old urchin at the Florence Nightingale Clinic on my first visit, was now going to Frank and Michele's school, started for sponsored orphans after they became frustrated with the poor education available. It had grown from a few classes, increasing every year as children went up to the next level. The school was fast gathering a reputation for the quality of the teaching.

Thomas was clean, polite and excited to see me. I gave him some new clothes and a plush gorilla that had been delivered to me in Adelaide by a member of the congregation at Westbourne Park whose grandson had decided to give his best toy to someone in Uganda. I knew straightaway it was for Thomas. His smile got bigger when I told him that, if he came to school on time every day for the term, he could keep the gorilla. He had only turned up for about half of the past term, so I was hoping the gorilla would inspire great things. Thomas's class sang me a welcome song. The teacher told me that when he arrived at this school he didn't know his letters, even though I had been paying for him to go to another school for two years.

Michele had brought Suzan to see me and she had grown quite tall and was animated and easy company. But her abdominal scarring was becoming very tight; Edward examined her and believed although previous surgery to the scars in her groin had allowed her to stand upright she would need more operations. It had always been a dream of mine to bring her to the Adelaide Women's and Children's Hospital to have all her scarring removed – without such a procedure she wouldn't develop breast tissue normally and could never have a child.

Bosco, once confined to a wheelchair, had improved dramatically and no longer needed the walking frame because he could manage with just a stick. His main problem was a urinary catheter which came out of his abdomen and drained into an old washing powder bucket. I wanted to get him a urinary drainage leg bag to lessen this indignity and later wrote home to see if Ruth Telfer at Resthaven could send some. I asked Bosco to clean and return his wheelchair to the hospital because he no longer needed it. Bosco had successfully applied for a micro-loan from UACO and set up a small roadside café with his wife, Aisha. She told me that her children no longer went to bed hungry and she could clothe them, put shoes on their feet and pay their school fees.

Tiny Noellina, who had been paralysed from the waist down, died while I was away. Florence reclaimed the bed that had been specially made for her by the hospital carpenter, and it wasn't long before we had a new use for it. On a walking clinic I met Godfrey, a paraplegic for fifteen years who slept on a mattress on the floor. We arranged for Noellina's old bed to be moved into his house, along with a back rest. Godfrey had two teenage daughters and a sister who lived nearby; his wife left him after the car accident that left him paralysed and was now dead. Although he had an old wheelchair, he never got out because he lived down a hill along a very bumpy road. There were already plans being made for a UACO celebration day toward the end of my stay and I invited Godfrey to come. It meant arranging special transport to bring him but everyone on the walking clinic was instantly excited.

There was a strange surprise one day when Recheal turned up to see me. I had been personally supporting her midwifery training since meeting her years before, but things had gone badly. While in Australia I received a letter from Recheal saying she was being poorly treated by the hospital administration staff and they were threatening to dismiss her. I wrote the medical superintendant an urgent email to find out what was happening. He replied that Recheal had lied about her name and qualifications. That plus her rudeness had led her to being sacked and I was devastated at the news. Despite all this, I still loved her and wanted to make sure she was alright. She arrived with her two-month-old son in her arms; there was an absentee father who sometimes saw him and gave her soap and washing powder. I reminded her of her past family planning lectures and she assured me that she didn't want to get pregnant again. She told me her mother had sold some land to pay for her to finish her training elsewhere. She had been accepted at another hospital and completed her certificate, and was now apparently a registered midwife and working in a clinic. In a way she had sorted herself out and seemed happy with her lot but I couldn't help wondering what else she could have achieved.

One night we received word that twelve piglets had been born to the two sows. They had both farrowed in one night and we had two very happy widows. It was so exciting to see the impact that the project could have on people's lives, especially those who had never experienced having money. The joy of piglets was to be shared: from each litter, the pig owner must give one piglet to someone who has nothing, and the only cost to that person is that when their pig grows and farrows, they must do the same. The loan recipients elected a supervisory committee from among themselves that visited each person with a loan every month to see how they were going. Bukenya organised a seminar on how to manage their money and used the language of the poor, not accountant-speak.

One of those with a piggery loan was Ritah, chair of the Najjanankumbi widows group. She had given a lot of input to the start of the group and during one of their regular meetings she spoke passionately about what UACO had done for her and other members. After the meeting and in recognition of her hard work, I told Ritah that UACO would help to fix her pig shed. She praised God and thanked us and then pleaded for me to go to her church so the pastors could bless me. This wasn't the first time she had asked me to do so, but for some reason I had always resisted and continued to. I was to find out why before long.

Like the widows, the youth group was making progress with their loan. They made money from growing cabbages and maize, despite a few problems with the maize such as flooding, thieves and then the landowner requiring the block back. Next came the youth's ambitious piggery project for which we had found sponsors back in Australia, starting with ten piglets and a plan to breed until each of the twenty-nine members had one piglet. It was difficult for them all to have a pen at home so they extended the piggery to include several growing pens. When the pig was old enough they could each decide whether to sell or breed from it. One conundrum that emerged was that Muslims cannot keep pigs, so there was talk of switching to goats. When they asked for my advice I said they all had good heads for thinking through problems; it was not for me to tell them what they want or need.

The youth group had formed a drama group that included young men and women and they were doing great things in the community. They saw their role as educating the community through song, performance and dance, particularly the young people, about HIV/AIDS, STDs and unplanned pregnancies. My plan was that when the next container was emptied, it would provide them with a place to meet, watch television and play games – like a clubroom.

In addition to the micro-loans for piggeries, UACO had built its own large-scale communal piggery. It was a short walk from the hospital in the middle of the slums. Edward's idea was that it could serve as a demonstration project to show others. It cost about $1500 but was well made of wood with an iron roof and iron sides to protect the pigs from the prevailing weather. There was one large pen for the boar, three pens for the pregnant sows and a pen adjoining for the piglets when they were weaned. The open areas were fenced off with barbed wire to discourage thieves. The land had been loaned to UACO by a widow who was sharing a small pigpen next door with another widow, where each had a sow.

Although farming in Uganda is very different from Nairne in the Adelaide Hills where we had our farm, I was able to pass on some techniques. The widows were fascinated that I could pick up a piglet by one leg and it didn't squeal. The biggest lesson was showing the women how much extra work was involved to keep the runts alive. There were always going to be more deaths here than in an intensive piggery in a developed country, but it was important they made the most of their animals.

The women who borrowed money were making their repayments on time and the one per cent interest paid was being used to fund more UACO projects. The management of the loans seemed to be going like clockwork – almost. I had a growing unease about something the widows called their 'revolving fund' and became more uncomfortable when I couldn't see any paperwork for it. It turned out the only woman not repaying on time was Ritah, the chair of the Najjanankumbi widows group. After some investigation, I discovered the paperwork showed no record of Ritah borrowing 160,000 shillings (about A$120) in August 2003 and there hadn't been a single shilling repaid. This presented me with a major problem because I had told Ritah a few days earlier that, because of her hard work and commitment to UACO over the years, we would renovate her pig shed to the tune of 700,000 shillings (A$500).

A community celebration day for UACO had been planned long before my arrival and the day was almost upon us. I didn't want to have a difference of opinion with Ritah when she was involved in organising the day, so let it wait. In the lead-up to UACO day Rose had taken me shopping for an African dress. Unlike a *gomez*, an African dress can be worn in any country on the continent and are always brightly coloured. The driver, Charles, also became intimately involved in the shopping expedition, freely giving his opinion on style and material. They decided on a vivid royal blue with gold embroidery. Rose promised to keep it a secret and as she dropped me off reminded me to dress 'very, very smart' on the day.

I'm not sure whether it was my outfit or the anticipation of a party, but when the day arrived I received a riotous welcome at the clinic, with joyful calling and ululating. Despite being hot and very dusty, everyone involved with UACO was there. The widows looked glamorous in their bright dresses. Edward sent his car to bring the *jajas* who otherwise wouldn't have been able to make it from their houses. It seemed to be more than a hundred people including community, police and church leaders. Shelters had been erected and decorated with streamers and balloons. Formalities got under way with lots of welcoming speeches followed by brilliant singing and dancing from the drama group as well as the widows groups from Najjanankumbi and Masajja.

I was seated next to a Catholic nun called Sister Rose and on the other side was Ritah. Suddenly she vacated her seat, telling me that a pastor was going to sit next to me. This seemed odd and I immediately had an uneasy feeling about this man. He kept leaning into me and insisting I visit him, but when I finally told him I didn't have any spare time left before I returned to Australia he soon slipped away, confirming my thoughts that he was up to no good.

My speech was the last one made. Edward interpreted as I spoke for ten minutes, and then I asked Edward to sit down. Despite my nerves, I spoke for about five minutes in Luganda, after which the crowd erupted – it was a wonderful moment. The local television crew was there to record the events (we made it onto TV a few nights later), and President Museveni's regional district officer was promising all sorts of things.

After the speeches, a birthday cake was cut by four *jajas* and I joined the widows to distribute it. Without thinking, I took the plates one at a time and knelt before each of the *jajas* and

Godfrey (the paraplegic who we had recently met on a walking clinic) and offered them the food; in Uganda, this is how you give respect to someone who is old. The crowd heaved with emotion and I was swept up into their arms and thanked and blessed. I could not tell how many pictures were taken. Edward's driver, Charles, grabbed me into a hug – I thought he was going to kiss me. He kept repeating, 'Thank you, madame, thank you, madame.' A beautiful photo of this unexpected and moving instant appeared in the paper the next day.

That weekend, as I lay in bed exhausted from the activity, thunder crashed across the city and then came the wonderful sound of heavy rain falling.

For several days I pondered how to discuss Ritah's situation with Edward. When I finally did, I discovered he knew all about it and assured me she would honour her debt. My response was to insist she pay back the loan with back-dated interest. He was caught between a rock and a hard place because he had promised Ritah's dying husband that he would take care of her and the children; I honestly don't know how many people this lovely man is responsible for. Florence was mortified about the whole situation, especially that she hadn't told me of the 'revolving fund'. I discovered that every time a widow paid off a loan she automatically was given a new one and so the small loan scheme had become a revolving fund instead of being open to new applicants. We spoke for a long time, during which several other issues came to light, such as the fact that some women were passing themselves off as widows in an attempt to get loans. This mild form of corruption had to stop.

Ugandans are so polite that it is very difficult for them to put people in their place. As a *mzungu* who was leaving soon, it was easier for me to speak directly to those trying to rip off the system, so I suggested to Florence that I could make it clear how things would be done. She was so relieved and said Edward would be too, because he worried about Ritah but didn't want to get too involved.

When we met with Ritah she apologised, then we worked out how to restructure her loan. The upgrade of her piggery would still go ahead after the repayments began. We praised her work with the widows group over the past three years and, in a face-saving effort, suggested she stand down as chair and accept the honorary (but powerless) title of patron. She thought that was a wonderful idea.

After six busy weeks, my final days in Africa were frantic, as usual. Florence and I visited the Congolese refugees and found ten adults and twenty-one children living there this time. Some of the refugees had been resettled in Norway while others had moved into smaller accommodation because the owner wanted his house back. There had been some improvement in cleanliness and the smell, but the conditions were still appalling. They were grateful for the free medical treatment. I heard the horrific story of one fifteen-year-old boy who actually saw the rebels eat his mother and wondered how this dear child could possibly live with the memory of such an event.

The clinic was bustling and one day Edward saw over one hundred patients, plus at least fifty mothers and babies for immunisation. Each child was given a toy after getting their shots.

I wasn't feeling great and my left femur was aching, but I was determined to go on one last walking clinic before I left, despite heavy rain turning most of the tracks into bogs. It was worth the effort.

Sisi, the beautiful blind *jaja* who I have known since I started coming to Uganda, asked for a photo with me so that her grandchildren could talk about it with her. When I told her I was going home, Sisi very softly started singing a song about saying goodbye and how much she loved me. Then the widows with me, Ruth and Jane, softly joined in the singing and my eyes filled up to overflowing.

I found one *jaja* in a dreadful state – so bad I would call it abuse. She was sitting on the floor on a mattress covered with black plastic because she was incontinent. Demented and dirty, she had not been cared for in any way for several days. I finally found a seventeen-year-old granddaughter who was responsible for her care and told me she fed her three times a day, did her washing and bathed her every evening. I did what I call my 'Jesus in the temple' thing and told her she was lying. I said her father was to be told that Judy Nambatya said he was not honouring his mother and should be ashamed, and that if he didn't like what I had to say he could see me at the hospital. While I spoke, the two widows swept and washed the floor and the girl made her grandmother a cup of tea.

Afterwards I reported them to the village authority, known as an LC 1. In Uganda, each district has leaders with various titles, starting with LC 1 and moving up to LC 5. Each rank brings greater responsibility and importance. Everyone who wants to qualify for a loan must have their application form signed by the LC 1 to show they are known and resident of a village. Unknown to me the LC that I had spoken to had in fact asked us to call on this *jaja* at the UACO Day celebrations. It was important for the family to know they had been reported to the LC 1 so they will take better care of their *jaja*.

I went to a farmers' market and bought some food and other things for Anna-Mary and Beth, including a kilogram of meat. A few weeks earlier I had been awoken at seven o'clock one morning by a banging on the door – it was Beth, desperate to show me her school report. I was barely awake, but understood her well enough when she quietly and respectfully said, 'I haven't got a schoolbag.' They were so delighted with the food, new schoolbag and clothes I had brought that they decided to host a 'meat party' that evening inviting their neighbours to share the meal. Beth read several verses from a Bible which I had given her three years ago and was now well worn. I wasn't convinced she had the academic ability to go much further than primary school, but Allan and I were committed to sponsoring her until she at least had a trade like sewing so she could earn an income. The room they lived in was so much better than their last, but it was still a slum which leaked when it rained and where rats gnawed the strap of Beth's shoes. The number of people living in the room varied from three to seven, depending on circumstances.

Everybody in Uganda needs so much that it can be hard at times not to take it personally. My final meeting with the youth group turned into a bit of a lecture from me about not always wanting. Instead we worked on ideas for income generation and what they could give back to their community. At the end of the meeting they announced that a special football match had been arranged in my honour the following Sunday afternoon.

In true Ugandan fashion, when we arrived for kick-off another match was being played. Eventually the teams agreed they would only play two thirty-minute sessions because it was going to get dark by 7 pm. At one stage a man pushed his wheelbarrow full of *matoke* across the pitch to save himself going all the way round, while another man rode his bicycle across, a cow following behind him. As it turned out, the first session went for thirty minutes and the second for fifty minutes; it appeared that the referee was the coach of the other team and, because the score was one all, he kept extending the match in the hope his team would boot another goal. Eventually he had to blow his whistle because it was almost too dark to see.

After long discussions with Edward, Florence, Bukenya and Ronald, we agreed they would form a management committee which met monthly and emailed me the minutes. The system would take some pressure off Edward so he didn't have to make all the decisions. The budget from Australian donations for the next financial year was over $18,000 and included an increase in Florence's salary.

On my last weekend, Florence invited me to her house for lunch and to meet her husband, Dan. He is a doctor and works about four hours from Kampala so is only home on weekends. I could tell he and Florence have a lovely relationship – they look as though they are very much in love. It is the same with Edward and Rose and it is special. I haven't seen that very much in Uganda.

My final presentation was always going to be emotional, but there was extra significance as we met in the Nigel Ambler Memorial Conference Room, which was packed to overflowing. I used prepared overheads to speak about successes and areas that could be improved. I then explained the structure of UACO, how we raised money and who got paid. It was a sharp reminder of how much is done by people for nothing: everyone involved with UACO was a volunteer with the exception of Bukenya, who is paid by Edward, and Florence and Ronald, who are paid by UACO. The other hospital staff are paid by Edward. There were needs everywhere, but priorities for now were rehabilitation facilities for the physiotherapist and another container of medical supplies for the hospital.

I was happy with how the meeting had concluded, but I should have known some more speeches and gift-giving were coming. I was holding it together until the youth group leaders, Ronnie and Paul, spoke. They told me that of all the things I had taught them, the most important was to love one another.

Then, one by one, the widows came up to say goodbye and they were all crying, as was Florence. Usually Ugandans are so strong and there is even a word in their language – *ngolabye* – which means 'do not cry'. Later, when I went to write my journal, the tears continued to splash onto the keyboard. All I could write was: *What a gift to be loved so much*.

Chapter Nineteen

ONCE AGAIN I RETURNED home via England to see Fiona and her family, then Allan and I travelled to Brisbane and Sydney to catch up with the boys and their families. It gave us time to talk and we returned home brimming with ideas about the people of Najjanankumbi. The challenge was finding enough money to do everything we wanted to.

Allan and Fred had started collecting rehabilitation equipment from various hospitals and organisations. It got busier for them after Edward wrote to the then South Australian health minister Lea Stevens asking for help with specific items. She responded that the government would be happy to give some surplus hospital and medical equipment, so for weeks the pair shuttled around South Australia collecting items from major Adelaide hospitals and regional clinics.

The wish list had started growing even while I was in Uganda. Lubega, our physiotherapist, told me of a three-year-old boy he was treating named Ssematimba Isham who has cerebral palsy. They needed a wheelchair for him because he was getting heavy and his body often went into spasm, making it difficult to carry him. Lubega hoped that when the child turned eight he could go to a special school for children with disabilities. I had emailed Allan to see if he could find a small wheelchair and my plea was met tenfold by a wonderful assortment of surplus equipment donated by Novita Children's Services (formerly the Crippled Children's Association). This would enable mothers of disabled children to get them out of their homes and into the sunshine and our rehabilitation clinic.

Once again the Kiwanis Club of Adelaide came to our aid and not only bought the six-metre shipping container we required but painted it inside and out as well. I had been debating the best way to use the container once it arrived, originally considering turning it into a flat where I could stay when in Uganda. However Kampala is such a noisy city and there is a loud night-time bar near the hospital compound which would prohibit any peaceful evenings. Eventually we decided it would become the medical clinic while the original container would become a multipurpose room rather than just a club room for the youth group.

By October 2004, the container was ready to be packed. We celebrated at Westbourne Park Church with supporters, some of whom had helped store equipment in their garages. Some returned on packing day to help the professionals. At the end we had some items left over and were able to give them to another organisation that regularly sent humanitarian aid to Africa.

While the emphasis of the first container was on furnishing and equipping the hospital, the second container was designed to help with small medical and consumable items, as well as containing dental and physiotherapy equipment. After the packing was done, an invoice was written up for customs:

205 cartons of consumable medical, hospital, physiotherapy, rehabilitation and clinic supplies
11 walking frames
1 hospital privacy screen
1 medical examination lamp
9 hospital beds
12 MediFlex hospital mattresses
2 medical/physiotherapy examination tables
2 hydraulic hospital trolleys
14 pairs of crutches
2 stainless steel children's hospital cots
2 stainless steel jugs
10 stainless steel hospital utensils
2 hospital bed lifters
1 blanket frame
5 IV stands
4 quad walking sticks
4 leg splints
31 walking sticks
2 pick-up sticks for disabled patients
2 lead X-ray protection coats
16 hospital sheets

48 hospital gowns

20 surgical gowns

29 hospital bedspreads

20 theatre tunics

308 theatre drapes

41 doctor's surgical trousers

8 MediFlex bolsters for physiotherapy

1 pair of adjustable parallel rehabilitation bars

1 child rehabilitation exercise machine

1 stationary exercise bike

12 exercise mats

2 child rehabilitation carry seats for cerebral palsy

3 child wheelchairs

5 child pushers

2 child chairs for clinic

10 boxes of educational resources

10 adult wheelchairs

1 trolley for transporting oxygen cylinders

13 chairs for clinic use

1 microwave oven for hospital/clinic use

1 complete set of doctor's surgical instruments

1 clinic ceiling ventilator

1 door and window and vent assembly for installation in clinic

1 box ultrasound gel

4 folding clinic tables

2 cans of clinic heat guard paint

As it sailed from Adelaide's Outer Harbour for Uganda via Singapore and Mombasa, I hoped the container would arrive as a Christmas present for Edward. Deep down though I was just hoping that it would arrive at all, given the notorious 1000-kilometre cross-country journey it would take from Kenya to Uganda, where looting is common.

Our prayers were answered (only four days late) and on 29 December the container was delivered to Najjanankumbi. Edward arranged for a cameraman to film the excitement for us to share. He wrote saying the quality of the equipment was better than anything he had seen in Uganda and he was amazed at the generosity of Australians. The unloading was like no other Christmas at Busabala Road, with the contents eliciting shrieks of joy. Lubega couldn't contain his excitement at the physiotherapy equipment and immediately used one of the small wheelchairs to help Ssematimba Isham. It was an instant relief to his mama, who had had to carry him for more than a kilometre to the clinic for treatment. Edward had organised a concrete platform for the container and it was placed at a right angle to the other container. Soon doors and windows were installed and a roof built to protect it from the weather. The UACO outreach was now 50 per cent bigger and could accommodate a meeting place for the youth, widow and HIV/AIDS groups, plus private counselling rooms.

About the same time, the management committee reported via email that a further twenty-three loans had been approved. On average, each loan was $230, which was more than double the first round. Our confidence in expanding the scheme stemmed from the success of that first round, when all the loans had been repaid. This is a well-known trend across the developing world – where micro-loans are given to women they have a stunning rate of repayment – and Uganda was no different.

One HIV patient with three children used a small loan to buy and sell *matoke* on the roadside; within months she had repaid the loan and borrowed three times the amount to expand her business to include a piggery. Now that she could afford the fees, her children were back at school. Another set up a small grocery shop to sell chapatis, while another widow with five children was selling charcoal and *matoke*. This was beneficial to those who had started businesses and also to UACO, as the interest received was a further step toward self-sufficiency.

The literacy program had also begun thanks to the generosity of a Janet Sutherland from Perth whom I had never met but who believed in the power of education. After hearing about UACO, she sent an email to Fred saying that she was asking guests at her fortieth birthday party to give a donation. It resulted in almost $1000 being sent. When asked if there was a specific program she would like the money directed toward, she answered that as a migrant who had arrived from South Africa a decade ago, the idea of funding a literacy school sat well with her. She has continued to support the project year after year, even as the cost of running the school tripled with the increase in students.

Eight students enrolled in the first course, committing themselves to three days tuition per week for nine months. The course began with reading, writing and numeracy and then branched into health lessons and civic education.

In a sign of growing respect for UACO, in 2004 the Ugandan Ministry of Health declared the clinic a designated immunisation area, which meant the government supplied the materials and UACO carried out the work. The government targets eight killer diseases: diphtheria, whooping cough, measles, hepatitis B, influenza, polio, tetanus and tuberculosis. At the same time we focused on diarrhoeal disease, nutrition, sanitation and hygiene (which included de-worming and vitamins). The result was 3000 children from nearby schools coming to the clinic.

That Christmas Fiona introduced Warrick to Australia and her Aussie friends, and we held a special blessing for baby John in the garden of our house. It was an opportunity for all of our friends and relatives to meet this new little family.

However amid the excitement of family reunions and the successes of UACO came an unexpected turn that forced me to rethink my work. It was late in 2004 when I was diagnosed with Parkinson's disease, a degenerative disorder of the nervous system that can take a toll on coordination and speech. I certainly had noticed a significant tremor, which got a lot worse when I was tired. The diagnosis was a shock and upset me for a while, especially as I feared major lifestyle changes including not being able to return to Uganda, as Parkinson's is a chronic and degenerative condition with no cure.

After a while I decided to just get on with life and not take too much notice of it. I had two dear friends who were significantly worse than me with this disease and I thanked God that mine was manageable for now – no two people are affected by it in the same way. But I was forced to review my lifestyle and decided my next visit to Uganda would be only six weeks rather than the three months I was considering. I began to wonder too how many more times I could visit Africa.

In the new year Allan and I headed off in the caravan for a few months on an extended getaway. We headed north from Adelaide via Alice Springs, and then on to Queensland along the Barkley Highway. We ate barramundi in Karumba on the Gulf of Carpentaria and camped by waterholes and rivers where we could hear the fish jumping at night. We left the van behind for a couple of days at Mount Carbine north of Mareeba to travel to Cooktown and then down the coast on a four-wheel drive track in the beautiful Daintree National Park.

Along the way I was devastated to learn that my dearest friend, Tanya Page, had died suddenly and unexpectedly. We had been work colleagues, friends and confidantes for years. It was so hard not to be able to go to the funeral but it was impossible to get back to Adelaide in time. I have missed her every day since. I think I always will.

We had only been back in Adelaide for one day when we were on the move again, this time in a different way. Several years before we had sold our holiday home at Port Elliot and bought the camper trailer. Allan and I had talked about selling our house in the city and moving permanently to Port Elliot, and then we learned about a house for sale there. Generations of Allan's family had holidayed in Port Elliot since the 1880s and we had continued the tradition; from an early age our children had gone digging for cockles in the surf and fished off the jetties. We bought the house at Port Elliot and sold our home in Adelaide very quickly. The house was thirty years old and very small so, although we were in theory downsizing, we planned an extension. Peter and Katrina were increasing the size of their family with a fourth child in August, so we'd need some room for visitors.

Amid the move, I was thrilled to be notified by the Zonta Club of Adelaide Torrens that they had awarded me their Woman of Achievement Award, in recognition particularly of the micro-loan scheme which had financially empowered many women. This was recognition of the work of many people, not just me, and I was delighted to receive it. Zonta is a service club for professional women, set up in America in 1919, which now has 1250 branches worldwide. In Australia, one of its projects is the provision of birthing kits for developing countries. The idea was formed in the Adelaide Hills where members had heard of its success in Nepal. After consulting with Anthony Radford, my teacher in international health, the group began packing basic medical supplies to help women who had little access to treatment during delivery. The kits cover what Anthony calls the 'seven cleans' of delivery: clean birth site, clean hands, clean ties (preventing bleeding from the umbilical cord), clean razor, clean gauze (to wipe the babies eyes clean of birth canal secretions and venereal disease germs before they enter the surface of the eyes, significantly decreasing infections), clean umbilical cord and clean perineum (birth area). He likes to add an eighth – a clean heart. What all that boils down to is a kit containing a square metre of black plastic, one scalpel blade, gloves, soap, three gauze swabs and two umbilical tapes.

The Australian Government aid agency AusAID funds the kits dollar for dollar with Zonta, and after being packed by volunteers they work out at a cost of just sixty-five cents each. In the late 1990s, the World Health Organization estimated that more than half a million women died annually in childbirth, 99 per cent of whom were in developing countries. For every woman who dies in childbirth there are another thirty who incur injuries and infections which can often be painful, disabling and embarrassing for life. Sixty million babies per year are delivered by a traditional birth attendant or with no assistance at all: this is the way the majority of babies are delivered in rural Uganda. UACO had become the Ugandan distribution centre for these kits and would eventually deliver thousands of Zonta birthing kits to remote clinics.

We were delighted with the move to Port Elliot and soon made wonderful friends at the Uniting Church there. In addition, Allan's sister Margaret and her husband Jeff retired from Sydney to nearby Victor Harbor. I loved the southern ocean coastline and walking Annie there every day. Sometimes we would see sea lions visiting from Kangaroo Island sunning themselves on rocks or surfing. I took photos on my new digital camera to show Edward and Rose what my new home and Australian village looked like. My mind easily drifted to Africa wondering how the projects were going. This was an important time for reflection.

The day before I left for Africa was a frosty morning and Allan and I drove along the esplanade so I could deeply breathe in the sea air and take it with me. This time I would be away for eight weeks in total, six weeks in Uganda and two weeks in London to visit Fiona, Warwick and John.

As I headed off, Allan was left living in our house while it was pulled down and rebuilt around him. I think I was getting the better part of the deal by living in a hostel in Uganda. At least I had a toilet and a shower – Allan often had to go to friends for one.

Chapter Twenty

THE PLANE TO KAMPALA was packed and as usual mine was one of only a few white faces. That would change a little in the next few weeks with three Australian women joining me in Uganda: Iva Quarisa, the daughter of our supporters and friends the Quarisas in Griffith; Sandy Lee, a radiographer from Sydney; and Viv Maskill, a registered nurse from Melbourne, who had heard about UACO and wanted to help and learn where they could.

Waiting at Entebbe were Edward, Rose and little Judy, who was now six years old. They introduced me to Frank, their new driver – I was shattered to learn that their previous driver, Charles, had been diagnosed with HIV/AIDS and taken his own life. Edward had loved him like a brother and missed him dearly.

The country was still tense after the turbulent general election a few months earlier that had seen President Museveni returned to office. It was the first multi-party election held for twenty-five years and there was plenty of bad blood between the six candidates. The main opposition leader, Kizza Besigye, used to be Museveni's doctor and fought in the bush war alongside him until he grew disillusioned and now led the Forum for Democratic Change.

Shortly after the election was announced, Besigye was arrested for treason and rape. He was accused of being connected to the brutal Lord's Resistance Army, a rebel group operating in the north of the country. His arrest resulted in riots, demonstrations and looting. At least one demonstrator was shot dead by police and Edward had to treat many casualties because the fighting was heavy near the hospital. An opposition office near the Busabala Road Hospital was frequently targeted and many were injured. Edward was grateful for the fence and barbed wire around the compound.

Museveni won the election with 59 per cent of the popular vote to 37 per cent, but Dr Besigye challenged the result, alleging it was fraudulent. The police had to use tear gas to disperse opposition supporters in Kampala.

In addition to the political upheavals, Uganda had been hit by a serious drought and water levels had fallen in Lake Victoria. This had affected the hydro-electric scheme and supply was a problem. Now when the power went off it usually stayed off for twelve to twenty-four hours.

The roads were constantly chaotic. Several nights I was awoken by car accidents outside the hostel and the city's tension grew with the frustration of deteriorating road conditions. On top of that, a lot of the extra traffic snarls were caused by preparations for the Commonwealth Heads of Government Meeting (CHOGM), scheduled to be held in Kampala in a year's time. New hotels were being built and old ones upgraded. Anywhere Queen Elizabeth would be driven was being fixed, and I was told any buildings on her route not finished in time would be bulldozed. It was hard not to think how much better it would be to put the effort into clean drinking water.

There was much news to catch up on and many people to see. I was thrilled to finally meet the new clinic administrator, Persis Kanabi Nsubuga, who had replaced Florence when she left to take up a position with the HIV/AIDS charity Mildmay. Persis was very gentle and quietly spoken. Although she was sixty-five years old, she looked fifteen years younger. It was exciting to have her working for UACO especially with her experience in development, small loan schemes and nursing. She hadn't worked for a long time but had returned to work after her husband died of cancer four years before. She lived on an acre of land, most of which was under some kind of food production including about 150 chickens.

The clinic needed immediate maintenance to fix the baby scales and the water tank used for inside hand-washing. The babies were being weighed on ordinary scales using a complicated system: first the mama held the baby and stood on the scales, then she gave the baby to someone else and was weighed again. The baby's weight was recorded by subtracting one from the other. It was easier to fix the scales.

Sandy Lee arrived the week following me after three weeks working in Rwanda. As a radiographer, she was part of a cardiac team called Operation Open Heart which functioned out of the Adventist Hospital in Sydney, each member volunteering their skills to provide cardiac surgery in areas of need. She was in her late twenties and planned to stay a fortnight in Uganda. When Edward and I picked her up from the airport she looked desperately tired and it turned out she was quite unwell. Soon after that, Iva Quarisa arrived in Kampala and they both joined me at the clinic.

Sandy and Iva were amazed at the dozens of mothers and their babies lining up for immunisation. Compared to what she had seen in Rwanda, Sandy was impressed with the hospital but to me it looked in need of a coat of paint. Edward had upgraded the maternity house to include two bedrooms, a lounge room and bathroom. He had also spent a lot of his own money demolishing and then rebuilding the physiotherapy area. When I went to have a look there was a great kerfuffle and I was shooed away and told I wasn't allowed to see it until the formal opening in a week.

Some of the youths came to greet me, but in reality they were more interested in speaking with my two young friends. It was funny watching them jostling for positions and flirting. When they found out Iva was going to play volleyball with them they were beside themselves. Iva had brought soft balls with her to teach the kids how to juggle; she'd really put a lot of thought into what she packed in her suitcase. The young people loved her and I later felt sure that of all the people who had visited UACO, she would be back. She has a real heart for helping young ones.

Iva confessed she was a little anxious when she arrived in Africa. I promised her parents I'd look after her but the three weeks she spent in Uganda were a steep learning curve – starting with a full clinic day and then venturing out into the community. The first walking clinic was full of shouting and joy. It was true to say that many of the people I introduced to Iva and Sandy were only alive because of UACO: previously there had been no services for them and many were in such a state they would barely leave their houses.

The last of my *mzungu* team arrived exhausted after flying from Melbourne to Kampala via Singapore, Dubai, Addis Ababa and Nairobi. Viv Maskill was a midwife who had also completed Anthony Radford's international health and medicine course; it was after I spoke to her student group about UACO that she enquired about visiting us in Uganda. Over the next two weeks she joined in every aspect of the outreach, including her particular interest of maternity. Although she missed two deliveries, she helped with the postnatal care – including watching the mothers climb on the back of a *boda-boda*, hanging onto their babies within hours of delivery for their ride home.

Bosco was delighted to have his urinary drainage leg bag but was desperately in need of more. He had been wearing his last one for months and it was dirty and blood-stained; I wrote to

Allan asking him to send some. Bosco needed some work for both income and self-esteem: the café he and his wife, Aisha, had started with a micro-loan was no more, as the owner of the area they had used for it wanted to build a shop there. The family was all very thin and now had no way of repaying the loan.

While we were visiting them we came across a tiny baby boy who had been abandoned and was being cared for by a lady nearby. Ronald, the nurse, came along on the walking clinics and agreed to provide follow-up care but, in the meantime, the baby didn't have a name. They asked me to think of one so I named him after my first-born grandson, Michael. I looked out for him at immunisation the next Tuesday and worked on a plan for him to survive. Sandy and Iva were challenged by what they saw on the walking clinic. They were like magnets to the children who followed them, running up to touch them and then race away to hide. Iva had handed out balloons and sweets she had brought from home. I wasn't sure who enjoyed it more, the Australians or the village children.

A few weeks later at the clinic I was asking about baby Michael when everyone smiled a little sheepishly. It turned out the name should have been Michelle, not Michael. Ruth, the woman who had adopted her, already had a seven-month-old baby but was happy to keep Michelle too. We tried teaching Ruth to breastfeed both but she resisted this, so we supplied her with formula.

The clinic figures gave a comprehensive snapshot of the health needs of the community. In the past twelve months almost 1000 patients had been treated, a third of whom were children under the age of five. Over 700 babies and children had been immunised. Gastroenteritis remained a huge problem with 75 per cent of the children reporting to the clinic being affected by it. There was also an outbreak of measles, and peptic ulcers and skin diseases were also a problem. Many conditions that wouldn't be a concern in Australia become very serious because of poor hygiene and malnutrition.

Among adults, poor nutrition and the stress of poverty led to cases of anaemia, hypertension, arthritis, infections, worms and malnutrition. There were many cases of sexually transmitted diseases, asthma and typhoid. But still the most common complaints were those resulting from HIV/AIDS patients who had infections, herpes, skin cancers, tuberculosis, chronic fever and coughs, all as a result of their immune systems slowly breaking down.

Each day as we drove down Busabala Road to the clinic, we passed successful projects as the result of small loans. One was a chapati stall made of sheets of corrugated iron which served the best I had ever eaten. Owned by a widow named Aisha, her two sons worked at the back of the stall, rolling the dough into lumps the size of tennis balls. They would then roll them out before putting them on a hotplate shaped like a shallow wok. After adding a little oil, a wad of newspaper was used to flatten them down while they were cooking. As well as the best chapatis around, they also sold charcoal to use as a cooking fuel. The business seemed to be going very well with a steady stream of customers.

Hadijah was another widow who was caring for seven grandchildren. She owned her own house and a bit of land where she had built quite a big stall to use as a warehouse, buying *matoke* in large amounts and then on-selling it to other stallholders. Robina was another AIDS widow selling *matoke* and vegetables in a small way, while Sofia sold charcoal and *matoke*. She also had a cow that was producing about three litres of milk per day; her business was going so well that she soon declared she was now 'in the middle classes'.

I developed a good working relationship with Persis and Ronald. Persis had a huge task as social worker, being responsible for community development, education and managing projects. She had a beautiful way with people, always being sensitive in her dealings with others. In his role as clinic nurse, Ronald was much loved by everyone, especially the elderly. In addition to running the clinic, Ronald counselled the HIV/AIDS and youth groups. At just twenty-seven, his maturity and commitment were amazing. As well as being a fully trained enrolled nurse and midwife, he had a diploma in HIV/AIDS counselling and was studying for a diploma in child psychotherapy so he could better manage the problems of the youth. He worked three half-days a week in the clinic and went to university in his time off.

Ronald's commitment to helping others came from his own family experiences. His father was killed in the Obote bush war and his mother died of AIDS. Ronald was harsh on himself for not having been there to help his mother, and this guilt manifested itself into a career caring for others with HIV/AIDS. His grandmother still lived outside Kampala but, because he could rarely get to see her, he found taking care of old people on the walking clinic reminded him of her. He was paying for the education his two younger siblings and helping his older sister through university. During one busy day he remarked that soon we will need to have UACO open five days a week. There certainly was the need, and he wasn't the only one who wanted it to happen.

Chapter Twenty-One

AFTER A WEEK IN Uganda I was formally welcomed back with a ceremony at the clinic. Wearing my blue African dress, I arrived at the hospital compound to find more than 200 people crammed onto the clinic verandah. Immediately there was shouting and cheering, and then each group presented songs, dances and poems.

First three little Congolese refugee girls recited a poem about war and sang a song, and then four boys sang and danced. The HIV/AIDS group nearly undid me with their wonderful singing and dancing. The leader, Pauline, is so beautiful and danced as gracefully as a gazelle. She knelt before me and sang and my eyes filled with tears. Then came the widows group and I really couldn't stop the tears. In no time they had me and the others up and dancing, and then they got Edward up too. I had never seen him dance before.

Iva, Sandy and Viv were welcomed too. Living all together at the hostel had been great. At the end of long days we would often just make toast with Vegemite and heat a cup of soup for supper, both because it was easy and because, in the two years I had been away, prices had shot up for accommodation, food and fuel. Edward and Rose were generous hosts. Each day Rose would make lunch for all four of us and Edward refused to take any payment, saying his culture did not allow it. Eventually I managed to get him to accept some money for fuel by telling him that UACO in Australia insisted.

It wasn't all work and we had a day trip to Jinja. The girls were snapping away with their cameras as we passed through tea and sugar plantations. Iva was particularly interested, given her work with the New South Wales Department of Primary Industries. She wrote up notes and became a kind of foreign correspondent for the department, sending back reports on how things were done in Uganda.

Iva was great company, very down-to-earth and practical, and I found we thought alike on many things. Like her parents, Iva loved people and would sit and listen intently to their stories, whether inspiring or heartbreaking. She wanted to help people and to see how they progressed. Although she only had a first aid certificate, she quickly absorbed the work of the clinic. Being a farmer's daughter, she was also particularly interested in the loan schemes that had resulted in small farms and agricultural projects. It became clear – to me if not Iva – that this wasn't a one-off interest.

It was obvious after meeting with the loan recipients that we needed to revise the rules. In my absence a committee of widows had been formed but no-one took responsibility for the money in an organised way so I suggested that we change the committee to include Bukenya and two HIV/AIDS victims, so that everyone had a voice in all decision-making. We decided anyone applying for a loan must prove they were local residents so the money helped the community, and later the rules were modified so that a person had to be registered with UACO for one year before applying for a loan, to stop those trying to get money without being committed to the community. And it was agreed small loans would be available for the poorest of the poor as a stepping stone to borrowing more.

Things became a little tense when concerns were voiced that Bosco and Aisha had outstanding loans. It was a difficult situation because I wanted to instil a discipline about repaying loans and not make UACO a welfare agency, but also to show compassion for these people. I told the group how I had taken the story of Aisha's café around Australia and inspired people to help. Through no fault of their own they had lost the café, and now both Aisha and Bosco were depressed and malnourished. Then I told them that after discussing it with Edward, Persis and the committee in Australia, I was wiping off the debt and they went ballistic, the air filling with 'Hallelujah' and 'Praise the Lord'.

The situation with Bosco was entirely different to the one faced with Ritah. She had the resources to pay back her loan but didn't and often disappeared for weeks on end. When I spoke with her about the two cases she accepted what had happened.

Persis and I gave Bosco the good news. In addition to clearing his debt we offered him a grant to get started again, and his face lit up like the sun. Bosco wanted to use the materials left from the first café to rebuild on a new site, but he was too weak to even nail the wood together so he started coming to the physiotherapy department to develop strength in his torso. It was then that I found that along with his multiple fractures at the time of his accident, he had broken his collarbone and it had healed badly and was subsequently weak.

Once they had their café up and running again, Aisha bought fish and sold it along with tea at her new premises. Soon she was making enough profit to pay her bills and look after the family. The difference in Bosco and Aisha's attitude was wonderful. They had a purpose again.

The HIV/AIDS group took out a micro-loan to begin a craft business, making woven mats, food containers, paper beads, crocheted baby rugs and handbags. They sold them at roadside stalls and community meetings where they also spread the anti-AIDS message, and they found ready buyers in Iva, Sandy and Viv. There were now sixty registered members of the HIV/AIDS group. They had many ideas and requests, including a bigger place to meet because the container was far too small for their growing numbers, and t-shirts to wear when they went into the community so others would recognise where they have come from. Many of the original members had died and five were now too sick to come to the clinic so were included in the walking clinic.

Life in Uganda was as difficult as ever for those with HIV/AIDS. Discrimination and denial remained high, especially in marriages and the workplace. Employees with AIDS were immediately sacked, and poverty and hunger were rife among sufferers. This of course created a vicious cycle, as without a strong diet the body weakens and gives way to the opportunistic infections which eventually lead to death.

A huge improvement could be made if the Ugandan Government supplied us with ARV (anti-retroviral) drugs that are commonly available to AIDS patients in the West. The drugs are not a cure but they strengthen the immune system when diet, hygiene and other basics are not a given, so conditions like tuberculosis, pneumonia and diarrhoea can be fought off. With this treatment, patients are able to live a relatively normal life, which is critical for families where an HIV-positive person is working.

Over the years I had visited Africa, the drugs had become available but while ARV drugs are free in Uganda, patients have to find the money for travel to major hospitals and large HIV/AIDS clinics, and even then the drugs may have run out when they arrive. If we at UACO could become a centre for distribution of the drugs the sufferer could be treated locally. I learnt though that in order to become a provider of ARV drugs we would need a special machine for the blood tests, which must be done prior to dispensing. The cost of the machine was roughly $55,000, well beyond our means.

While many of the HIV/AIDS group were successfully managing their loans, I soon had to tackle an awkward case when I discovered that the largest outstanding debt belonged to Ronnie, the previous leader of the youth group. He had been allowed to borrow far too much and wasn't able to make the repayments, but when we met to discuss his predicament he promised to make monthly repayments until he paid off what he owed. I believed him.

This sort of administrative work was increasing as gradually UACO moved from its infancy into an established institution. Although I went on walking clinics and visited the clinic, most of my time was spent going through reports and spreadsheets. Not everything needed to be put into the newsletters we put together for distribution back home, but the Australian supporters who had trusted us with money needed to know where it was being spent and with what effect.

One walking clinic was delayed by torrential rain. When we set off we were slipping and sliding under our umbrellas, trying to stay upright. We weren't always successful. I ended up on my backside quickly followed by Jane, one of the widows, and we dissolved into fits of laughter. By the time I got home I had to soak my shoes in a bowl of water and scrub them to get the mud out.

Despite the weather, we had many wonderful visits with old friends. The blind *jaja* Sisi was so happy we were there – she said she could tell it was me by my voice and the feel of my skin. We stopped in at youth group leader Paul's house, which he shared with his mother. His father died from gunshot wounds when Paul was three months old and his siblings were all dead from AIDS. There were about ten grandchildren, all of whom Paul and his mama were trying to educate. Paul had recently graduated from university with a degree in education, but like so many Ugandans with tertiary qualifications, as yet he had no job.

I was finding the walking clinics hard work physically. While parts of my body no longer wanted to go up and down steep hills the other part of me loved this side of UACO. It was so important to go deep into the villages looking for young mothers and babies needing immunisation. There was also a simple joy of village life. At every step something is happening. All the tiny shops are trading and food stall owners plying their wares. I was well known by now and the locals called out to me by either of the names that I have become known as '*Oliotya Nambatya*' or '*Oliotya* Mama Jude'. Translated it means 'Good morning how are you'.

Word was spreading of the work UACO was doing, and one day I walked into Edward's office to find two Catholic nuns from a maternity clinic a hundred kilometres away. They had heard about the Zonta birthing kits, of which Edward gave them 200, then they posed for a delightful photo for the Zonta Club.

Edward clearly explained to them that the kits were not to be sold and that they would need to report back to him on their use. Over the next few weeks the rest of the kits were distributed, and Edward put up a map on his office wall marking all the places they were being used.

After weeks of anticipation, the secret of the new facility at the hospital was revealed. I was taken to the hospital where, in true Ugandan style, a crowd had gathered, including representatives from the youths and widows. After speeches were made, Edward invited me to remove some paper off the wall revealing a sign underneath:

JUDY STEEL REHABILITATION CENTRE (PHYSIOTHERAPY)

I was speechless.

Edward had renovated and rebuilt the facility beautifully. There was an office, waiting room, tilt bed for postural drainage, ultrasound room, large exercise room, equipment room and two very large toilet rooms with sinks. Lubega took centre stage, taking nearly three hours to tell us in minute detail about every piece of equipment. He kept repeating, 'There is nothing like it in all of Uganda.'

Waiting out the front before the opening, I realised that the little boy with cerebral palsy who had needed the wheelchair was before me. He was growing well and his mother was obviously giving him the best care she possibly could. She sat next to me inside and while I stroked the little boy's face he smiled at me, and I was a little misty eyed when I realised the difference that was being made to the lives of this child and his mother.

To complete her Ugandan education, one morning I took Viv to the Florence Nightingale Clinic at Nakulabye to walk through the slums with me. In the brief time we were there I found Thomas and his mama; he was very quiet and as usual he needed a good scrub. When we returned home Viv was a little quieter than normal. Although we had been working in tough conditions in Najjanankumbi, things were worse in Nakulabye where the population was larger and the facilities at the Florence Nightingale Clinic more basic.

About a week later, Beth and her mother, Anna-Mary, came to Edward's hospital. Anna-Mary had had constant malaria which required medication via injection from time to time. Beth said she was having trouble at school but that her grades were fair. In truth her grades were terrible and she wasn't learning. Despite going to school, each night she would return to live in a one-room house with anything up to seven people there. Without a table to sit at or electricity to light the room she had no chance to study. It was very sobering because she had grown very tall and pretty but thin because of a lack of food.

Work at the UACO clinic continued and hundreds of mothers came to learn, with family planning top of the list. Ignorance of medical conditions was one thing, but so many women had no idea about their own bodies. One little mama came in with her six-week-old daughter. Just eighteen, she lived with her aunt but had a man who 'looked after' her. She had never heard about family planning and I told her she was too young to have another baby straightaway. She was grateful and came back for more information. Thankfully, others were getting the message. A Congolese refugee we knew as Mama Thomas had three children under five and, although she didn't speak English, she made me understand clearly that she was not having any more babies.

Edward was very worried about two teenage orphans. They were members of the youth group and beautiful dancers in the drama group, but Edward feared that they would be in real danger where they were living. He wanted to bring them to live in the hospital – there were some rooms in the old part where he housed young ones and supplied them with food and pocket money. In return, they cleaned the hospital before going to school. If they showed promise he trained them to be nursing assistants or helpers around the hospital. Iva stepped in and agreed to help the two girls through secondary school by paying their school fees.

I was sorry to see my three Aussie friends go. They had been great company and each evening we would gather in my room to discuss the day. They all left at different times, Sandy tried first but as she boarded the plane at Entebbe she started vomiting and eventually caught a taxi back to the hostel. We nursed her for several days, Edward arriving in the dark one night on a *boda-boda* to administer intravenous antibiotics. Viv left after two weeks for Zambia and Iva left last of all. She was the same age as Fiona and we had become great friends. In my heart I knew she would return to Africa.

Underpinning all of UACO's operation was Bukenya. In addition to being a fine accountant, he is a wonderful person who radiates love. He is a Muslim and his father had three wives but doesn't take any care of them or his children. Bukenya lived alone because his mother and some of his brothers lived in the country while a sister was going to university. Bukenya was only twenty-six years old but paid all their school and university fees.

Despite all his work, I still found auditing UACO a draining experience. The toughest part was finding a quiet space and a block of time when no-one was around – a bit like finding hen's teeth in Uganda. Often when I did find some spare time to start work, the power would go off and take computer access with it. One time I thought I'd found a nice quiet moment at the hostel until a group of girls arrived back from a school break and started screaming with delight as they caught up with each other. Soon after came the booming sound of dance music…

The UACO clinic was functioning within budget but the cost of drugs staggered me. The first time I looked at the receipts I thought we were covering the cost of the entire hospital, but that was just what basic medicines cost in this country. Edward buys in bulk to get the best price, but the growth of UACO was reflected in the ever-expanding pharmaceutical bill. During a conversation about the cost of things, Edward said he gets stressed when I am there because the community presumes that he gets paid millions by UACO. After that, whenever I spoke to groups of people I would go through the structure of UACO and emphasise who was paid and who wasn't, emphasising that Edward was a volunteer. This was a relief to him.

The generator was another major cost but was an essential for both the hospital and clinic given the constant power outages. It cost roughly $20 to run it for ten hours using twelve litres of diesel, and servicing it was an added expense. Although mostly reliable, it was still unpredictable. One day a power surge from the regular power supply blew up Edward's fax machine and only the surge arrestor stopped the computer suffering a similar fate.

My financial concerns about Ronnie had been sorted out, but the youth group continued to provide me with headaches. I was disappointed during our first meeting on this trip when they just wanted more, more and more. They asked for new uniforms, football boots, footballs, volleyballs, gardening tools and at least one wheelbarrow. Their only suggestions for self-improvement seemed to involve me buying them things. They had written a report of their activities explaining how they had been busy with community service, but I couldn't see any examples of it. The water well next to the hospital clearly hadn't been cleaned for a long time and there was a lot of rubbish around their piggery. We held another meeting during which I expressed my concerns, making it clear that I didn't want to be told things that were not true.

Then it was time to show, not tell. I took three young men from the group with me on a walking clinic and, at the end of it, Paul confessed he had had his eyes opened. We found one young mother without a husband. She was living with her very old grandmother, six children and one baby. As usual, the parents were all dead of AIDS and the mother had ended up with the responsibility of caring for them. I took the opportunity to teach my young friends that the birth of the young baby was the result of unsafe sex and the mother will in all probability have or get AIDS. The baby had only had one of his scheduled immunisations, but by the time we left she knew all about the correct immunisations for her baby, how to protect herself and where to come for information about family planning.

We went on, and I was sitting down in the dirt with a *jaja* cooking maize on a charcoal stove when we noticed a small child with matted hair. On closer inspection, I found his ear was pouring forth pus and he had secondary infections on his scalp. The poor little chap was in much pain. We found his mother and sternly insisted she bring him to the clinic.

After the walk, we talked about the experience and one of the youths named Ivan told me in broken English that he had learnt that *jajas* love you to love them, and you can hug them and they don't mind. Five gold stars for that boy. They promised that one of the youths would go on the walking clinic each week from then on. There is so much they can help with, like fetching water, washing clothes or cleaning up around the house.

Sadly, the UACO communal piggery was a disaster. We had invested roughly $750 building it and a similar amount stocking it with pigs for a return of about one-tenth of that from their sale. It wasn't in a good location and Edward and I agreed it had to go. We were able to recoup some money by selling the operation to the people who owned the land and originally shared the piggery. Edward used the returned money to buy plastic chairs. They are in short supply in Uganda and, given the country's love of speeches and formal events, they are highly sought after for hiring. The chairs provided a steady stream of income without fear of swine fever or lack of feed.

UACO's expenses continued to escalate and, in addition to the rising costs of drugs and fuel, we needed to find money to boost the pay for the key staff, Ronald and Persis. Both were struggling on the meagre amount we could afford, and yet they were so capable I couldn't imagine losing them. When Florence resigned, Edward interviewed four people for the position and Persis was the only one we could afford – none of the others would even consider the position for the salary offered. I shall love Persis forever for accepting the position. UACO was fast gaining a reputation as a dynamic organisation and attracting interest from medical people (Edward's colleagues often expressed envy at his hospital's equipment and facilities), but we were also getting a reputation for not paying enough. Persis had a lot of qualifications and experience aside from nursing. She was wise and lovely, she managed everyone calmly and quietly and they respected her very much. Although wages in Uganda are generally 10 per cent of those paid in Australia, on our current budget we could only manage about half that.

During our full executive meeting in the last days before I was due to leave again, we discussed the budget. Fred, in his role as treasurer, emailed approval for an overall increase, saying there was enough money from Australian donations to include a wage rise for both Ronald and Persis, which was wonderful to be able to announce. After the meeting the farewells started. They presented me with a beautiful *gomez* and Edward gave me a *kunzu* (traditional men's formal robe) for Allan.

I took Anna-Mary and Beth two big bagfuls of food and left money with Frank and Michele to buy Beth some new clothes at Christmas. Beth's latest school report was not good, and I talked with Frank and Michele about taking Beth out of school. She was now fourteen and had never been able to comprehend schoolwork. I suggested training her in something such as cooking, but the biggest fear at this age is that if she left school she would be at risk in the community and that it would be better for her to stay in school for another two years. A girl of fifteen is considered sexually active in Uganda and often at risk of prostitution. I feared Beth would be easy prey for this given her naivety and aimlessness.

I took an exhilarating *boda-boda* ride to visit Frank and Michele at their home in Lugala and Thomas came and showed me his schoolwork; he said his favourite subject was English. We had a lovely time and I told him I was very proud of his neat writing. He loved the new backpack and clothes I had bought him.

As always, my heart strings were being tugged by the time I had finished saying goodbye to everyone and I was feeling such a mixture of emotions. Glad to be finished and excited that I would soon be returning to a protein-filled diet with a glass or two of red, but also desperately sad that I wouldn't see my extended family for some time. I told Edward it would probably be three years before I returned, but he refused to hear that saying: 'No, no – I cannot do without you for more than two years.' I knew many of my beautiful friends would die before I came back.

Chapter Twenty-Two

AFTER LEAVING UGANDA I flew home the long way via California. Fiona and Warrick had moved to San Francisco and now had a baby girl named Katherine Eleanore, known as Kate. She just melted into my arms at the airport. John was a little more reticent but that soon changed. I spent all of June 2006 in heaven being a mum and a nanna. What a wonderful way to recover from the stresses and strains of working in Africa.

My time in San Francisco may have been peaceful but there was one particular weekend that was anything but for Allan back in South Australia. I had known for a few months that I was to be recognised in the Queen's Birthday Honours list by being appointed an Officer of the Order of Australia (AO), but the phones ran hot after the news broke on the June long weekend. Allan was on the phone continually dealing with our friends and the media. Once again I felt overwhelmed by this honour and truly believed it recognised the work of many people – Allan and I have often joked he should have received the Companion. I could never have done what I have done without his constant love, support and advice.

I arrived back from the States in time for us to be guests for the investiture at Government House in Adelaide, where I received the award from the governor of South Australia, Marjorie Jackson-Nelson. I also returned home to find the house largely rebuilt and extended and, although we lived in the caravan for a couple more weeks, things were moving along very nicely. Port Elliot is so tranquil, and walking along the coast with Annie was a perfect time for reflection. I have a special seat where I sit and talk to God, and the seals and the whales when they are visiting from the Antarctic.

I had not been home long when I learned that members of the Port Eliot Uniting Church had become very excited about UACO. Although essentially an older congregation, they supported it financially and keenly sought an update on Uganda.

The next instalment in the UACO story was an unexpected one. We had been trying to source an ambulance for a couple of years from different ambulance services around Australia, but nothing had eventuated. Anthony Radford was working at the Repatriation General Hospital in Adelaide when he noticed a couple of orderlies looking at a website that showed a picture of an ambulance. It turned out they were both weekend volunteers for St John Ambulance, and Anthony remarked that he was looking for an ambulance. They explained the organisation turns their vehicles over every ten years and there was in fact one outside for sale.

Within five minutes Anthony was on the phone to the chief executive of St John Ambulance Australia, Peter Gill, discussing the work of UACO and how badly an ambulance was needed in Uganda. The next day, St John offered one of their decommissioned vehicles to UACO at no cost. A mechanic, the son of a member of our congregation at Port Elliot, did a complete service and safety check of the ambulance. Another couple donated a significant portion of the cost of shipping the vehicle to Africa. We decided it would be a wasted opportunity if it was shipped over empty and so began again collecting medical supplies and consumables. They all came from pharmacies, organisations and individuals on the Fleurieu Peninsula south of Adelaide. By the time the 1996 Ford Econovan ambulance was driven into the shipping container, it was jammed full of:

- medical X-ray film
- incontinence pads
- dental instruments
- sterile cottonwool buds
- 15 walking sticks, 1 walking frame and 1 quad walker for physiotherapy use
- bandages
- urology–colostomy drainage items
- medical instruments, airways, infusion sets

combine dressings

surgical gloves

2 wheelchairs

tissue packs for clinic use

cotton-tipped probes

clinic and hospital soap

hospital covers and air cushions

nebuliser

breast pump

surgical items

neck braces

urinary catheters

urinary drainage systems

antibacterial wipes

emergency siren for ambulance

Once again a container-load of treasure was sent off to Uganda, but it wasn't long until it became entangled in a frustrating round of African bureaucracy. Edward and his driver, Frank, travelled to Mombasa in early December, intending to drive the ambulance the 1000 kilometres to Kampala. However, once there the Kenyan authorities decreed the vehicle was in transit and so couldn't be driven, and certainly not when loaded with medical supplies. The goods had to be unloaded, checked against the manifest and then repacked into the ambulance, which was then put back into the shipping container, re-sealed and sent to Kampala. A month after first arriving at Mombasa, the ambulance was finally parked in the hospital compound.

Our ambulance wasn't the only new transportation. I had spoken to a Probus group at Port Elliot about Ronald's workload, explaining how he frequently made urgent night visits to the elderly, mostly on foot. If we could get Ronald a *boda-boda* he could move quickly, particularly when someone with malaria needed an urgent intravenous infusion. A couple, Sue and Anthony Smith, approached me after the event offering not only to pay for one but also to cover the annual cost of maintenance and fuel. Ronald was soon well known throughout Najjanankumbi for his motorbike equipped with a box on the rear to carry medications.

Our son Peter was serving in Iraq for six months, leaving Katrina a sole parent taking care of their four sons, so Allan and I went to help out for a while in February 2007. The army posts Peter to a new place every two years and now the family were in Canberra. One of the things we have had to come to terms with is that if your children are in the defence forces then what you used to think was normal no longer is. When they joined we had no idea what terrorism would do to global security and how the role of the soldier would change to combat that. Peter was based in Basra and regularly went to Baghdad. I used to worry deeply about his safety but in the end decided that I had to trust him to God or I would have gone crazy. When he returned from that tour he was made Commanding Officer of 5 Aviation Regiment Townsville.

Our eldest son, David, and his wife, Jodi, were working hard to take magnificent care of Cameron, who was now six years old. Born with cystic fibrosis, he is now going to school and manages to not miss too many days. Very bright and inquisitive, which is often the way with children with cystic fibrosis, Cameron is a sensitive little boy who often sounds so much older than his years. His sister, Claire, three years younger, is full of mischief, love and laughter.

In early 2007 we were shocked by the news that Luigi had died in Griffith. Since that first meeting in 2000, the Quarisa family had been loyal supporters of UACO but were also now very dear friends. Luigi and Mary had been married fifty-four years. His daughter Lizabeth wrote a moving tribute to him:

My father was a modest man, who never wanted to be famous or the first. His schooling was brief but his education complete. And for me, he was the greatest man because he taught us always to do our best. To learn as much as possible about the world and to give to the very end. And if we have inherited even a part of his being, then this world will be a better place.

We were not surprised to be among hundreds who came to pay their respects. At the service mourners were asked to donate to UACO in lieu of flowers, and so came a final gift for Uganda from this dear man.

Almost every monthly report emailed from Uganda showed a growing need. The clinic operated two days per week but could have run five. In the year 2000, 564 babies were immunised but by 2007 that number had reached 3500, with a forecast it would top 5000 within twelve months. The number of clients receiving medical treatment and counselling for HIV/AIDS was expected to double in a year. The clinic's pharmaceutical bill was now almost $1000 per month and more than a quarter of the total annual budget. The micro-loan scheme was constrained by the funds available, with applications far outstripping approvals. The first group had graduated from the functional adult literacy class while the waiting list to enrol grew longer by the month. It all boiled down to simply not having the funds to support any expansion; as it was, we were barely covering the current level of services. Fundraising was sustained by regular generous donors but we were always looking for ways to find more money. Our search led us to apply to AusAID for a one-year grant.

AusAID, the agency that manages Australia's overseas aid, works out of the Department of Foreign Affairs and Trade in Canberra, but also has staff at various embassies around the globe. Its goal is to use the tens of millions of dollars it receives each year to reduce poverty and achieve sustainable development in line with Australia's national interest.

I found writing the proposal really complex and difficult, however, with the help of Allan, Fred, Iva and Edward and his team from Uganda, we applied successfully for $45,500 – enough money to expand the primary health care service into the slum areas adjacent to Najjanankumbi. AusAID grants do not pay for staff wages, rent or construction of buildings, but ours did allow us to buy medications, 600 mosquito nets and more food supplements for HIV/AIDS sufferers. It also allowed for an expansion of education programs that teach about malaria, STDs, family planning, literacy and how to manage a small loan.

The exciting news of the grant came as I prepared to return to Uganda. I decided that three years was too long to be away and I planned a nine week visit for early in 2008. There was so much to do this time with the implementation of the grant and Edward was anxious that I oversee everything. He was aware he had to show the Australian Government that he was honest and accountable for the 'model of community care' which was the title of our application.

Since I was last there, the Ugandan Government had banned plastic bags so I began collecting environmentally suitable shopping bags to take with me and soon had 250. These were packed alongside 150 knitted babies' garments, one hundred girls' dresses, thirty pocket teddy bears and twelve Adelaide Crows beanies for the youth group. We were also given three cardiac monitors and a defibrillator. A transport company shipped them from Adelaide to Brisbane free of charge where they were included as part of a larger container destined for Michele and Frank Heyward in Uganda.

On this visit I once again had an Aussie team coming, with Fred eager to meet Edward and all the people he had been interacting with over the years. Iva was returning for the second time and her friend Anthony Catanzariti from Sydney was eager to see what we do.

The long journey to Uganda began at 3.30 am when we pulled out of our driveway and headed up the dark and silent highway to Adelaide. It is always a time of both excitement and anxiety. I always miss Allan so much but I was worried about how my health would be this time, though my Parkinson's was relatively stable and hadn't changed much in the past year or two. I did have days when I felt quite shaky but I could generally manage well. This would be quite a test.

Chapter Twenty-Three

As usual, I had excess luggage consisting of three suitcases, laptop computer and carry-on bag. I was thrilled when Qantas checked it all through to South Africa for free. My good fortune didn't last though and, after an overnight stopover in Johannesburg, I returned to the airport and faced a penalty for thirty-three kilograms of excess baggage. The line at the service desk had taken so long people were kicking their luggage in frustration. I was quite stressed by the time I reached the front of the queue because my flight left in less than an hour, then for some reason the woman behind the desk started talking to a colleague rather than processing my ticket. I had to raise my voice to get her attention during which my Parkinson's really kicked in and both hands were shaking.

I made it to Uganda late that night and it was clear improvements had been made for CHOGM. The hotel in Entebbe where I stayed overnight had had an upgrade and I was delighted to have room service of soup and a toasted sandwich before collapsing into bed

Edward and Rose arrived the next day with little Judy to meet me. On the drive I was startled by the greenery. South Australia had suffered through a horrendously hot summer that had dried everything to a crisp, so to see green grass and water was a pleasant change. Edward said the rains had caused flooding in many houses in the low-lying areas with some loss of life. He warned me I would need rubber boots for the walking clinic.

I had decided to stay at a hotel that was walking distance from the hospital this time rather than the hostel. It looked great from the outside but my room consisted of a bed, small table and two chairs. The ensuite was a tiny room opened by a water-soaked plywood door with a nail as a handle. In the middle of the metre-square area was a toilet that didn't flush; instead I had to spray water from a hand-held shower hose into a bowl and toss it down. The bedroom was so small I couldn't unpack my belongings and had to sit the computer on my knees to use it. The first night, the noise was horrendous from the bars downstairs: the next morning a church service was held in the conference room next to mine which went for hours and hours, and by the end I knew both fifty different ways to say hallelujah and that I would have to stay somewhere else. Edward had thoughtfully not cancelled a booking he had made at the hostel in case I didn't like the hotel, and so the next day his driver, Frank, came around and helped me move.

After a huge welcome back from Bukenya and others at the hospital, Edward insisted I visit the rehabilitation centre, which was building a reputation as one of the better physiotherapy clinics in Kampala and being referred to patients from different parts of the city for treatment for back pain, cerebral palsy, fractures, dislocations and sports injuries. Although the centre is part of Edward's hospital and not part of UACO, we did equip the facility so UACO clients could be treated free of charge, thanks to income received from paying patients.

Once inside I was stunned to see Godfrey in his callipers and crutches moving haltingly across the room. The dear man was so determined to show me how he had progressed. Although he would never be able to properly walk he was able to move about, change his position and have some independence. He had also been able to get a small loan in conjunction with his sister and was selling charcoal at a roadside stall, but the previous Christmas he was struck down by a bad bout of malaria that claimed the life of his sister. Godfrey couldn't manage the business alone and so sold it off to clear his debt. He was now back on track and at forty-four years old was ready to rebuild his life. His chest and arms were very strong and he could now haul himself up on callipers that not only help him avoid the sort of morbid conditions that can occur being wheelchair-bound, but also drew him up to eye level with other adults and increased his self-esteem.

After the thrill of seeing Godfrey's progress came the big news that Bosco had had successful surgery to reconnect his urinary system making a catheter unnecessary, plus he had a small business and no longer needed a walking stick. I was overwhelmed at this outcome. Apparently Bosco was somehow sponsored to have his surgery and UACO paid for the X-rays. The only sad part of the story was that his wife, Aisha, had gone off with another man and had a baby. Two of Bosco's children were living with him and he had used a second small loan to set up a stall cooking and selling food, and on a good day he could earn four dollars. Edward told me many times that Godfrey and Bosco are the most successful stories of UACO and we must tell everyone about them.

The clinic was bubbling along but the rain had turned the area between the two containers into a bog, so over the next few weeks it was concreted. I was delighted to see one of the women from the literacy class working among the young mums, selling the soap she makes as the result of a small loan. She had the brightest personality and chatted easily, encouraging the mamas. Persis suggested developing a young mothers club as many knew little about raising a child, managing a crisis or just the normal day-to-day things that young mums need to talk about. With about 130 mothers aged between fourteen and twenty-two on the books, many uneducated and illiterate, it seemed a more than worthwhile idea. The project took off and within months we had 800 mothers coming to the clinic for mothers club meetings each month.

The literacy school was going so well that it needed to be expanded from two classes to three. The teacher, Paul Lutalo, had a degree in education and could have been employed in high schools but instead chose to work for UACO. Some of his students didn't even know how to hold a pencil when they came into his classroom. As the number of students grew, we needed to find the money to pay Paul more and hire an assistant or risk losing him. The classrooms were so tightly packed that he literally couldn't get around to help all the students individually, so we also needed more sessions to thin out the groups. There were suggestions too for a creche to take care of the little ones while their mothers were in class. As well as teaching the women and men to read and write, Paul brought in other UACO people to speak to the students about what they did, such as Herbert from rehabilitation, Bukenya from small loans, Persis, Edward and nurse Daniel Otieno, who was now full-time in the clinic.

Daniel had replaced Ronald, who left UACO to follow his heart. In 2006 a young nurse from Sydney named Lara Shelton spent six months in Uganda with UACO. While becoming a dynamic part of the outreach, she also fell in love with Ronald. They returned to Australia together and married, and Ronald began studying at university for his Bachelor of Nursing.

Daniel had been working for Edward in the Busabala Road Hospital and was a registered community nurse. It had long been a passion of his to work in the community setting so he moved across to the clinic. Born in Kenya to a Ugandan mother, his father had died and so Daniel was responsible for the education of his seven siblings. Despite this, his commitment to the clinic was extraordinary. One of the first things Daniel showed me was the *boda-boda* donated by Sue and Anthony, which he used on his evening runs.

Although basics like food and fuel were more expensive since my last visit, anti-retroviral drugs for the treatment of AIDS were more readily available. The Mildmay clinic was now offering blood tests and then cheap or even free drugs. Some AIDS victims we were seeing were getting these drugs and they made such a difference because they allowed those suffering from AIDS to lead a more normal life. However, Mildmay was several kilometres away and involved money for transport which most did not have.

At our first meeting I told everyone about receiving my award in the Order of Australia, explaining it was as much theirs as mine. They gave me a huge clap when they saw the photo. I also explained all about our AusAID grant, then shared my feelings of frustration and exclusion when in Australia by not hearing news such as ARVs becoming available and the youth drama/dance group coming first in their competition. It was really important to me that I didn't have to wait two years to find out.

When I finished, Edward gave the following summary of my talk and his reaction to it:

1. We must work as a team.
2. We must be ready to take on responsibility.
3. Australia has shown that they love us and we must show others that we love them. (I nearly cried at this point.)

4. Why should Judy be here? It is her love for us. (Nearly more tears.)
5. We should do things for the very poor.
6. This will lead to good governance because our youths are the future leaders of our country. If our youths learn about human rights and crime prevention they will become good leaders.

Over time, without noticing it, my relationship with Edward and Rose changed. By some bitter experiences of the past I was often mistrustful of Ugandans, but Edward was so different that I would trust him with my life. Often, when things boiled up in me I would go straight to him and he was always understanding and acted where he could. Most days I would have lunch with Edward and Rose, and Rose would ply me with mounds of Ugandan food such as *matoke*, chapati, fish or chicken and peanut sauce; she always said I was not to lose one kilogram while in Uganda. I really enjoyed those breaks with them. We understood each other's senses of humour better as the years went on and so often there were deep belly laughs over lunch.

The HIV/AIDS group had grown and now included many men. At our first meeting I was so proud of them when they reported that none of them had died in the time I had been away. One of the reasons they were so well was because of the food supplement being provided by the clinic in the form of a soy and millet porridge which was high in protein and carbohydrate.

One of the most enthusiastic was Pauline. A beautiful and confident woman, both she and her partner, Johnson, have AIDS. Pauline regularly volunteered in the community to spread the word about the disease. She would wear one of the special t-shirts provided by UACO to be easily identified and talk to anyone and everyone about how not to contract it and what to do if you had. She brought me to tears when I asked her why she had enrolled at the adult literacy class and she replied that she wanted to be able to write her own name before she died.

After one meeting, Pauline approached me and said she wanted to be married by a minister in a church before I left. I was so excited. We quickly agreed to host the reception at UACO in three weeks time. Her friends arranged to 'dress' the bride and with everyone at UACO contributing a small amount we would be able to pay for some samosas, soft drinks and a wedding cake.

Frank had been working as Edward's driver for three years. A small man in his late twenties with a beautiful gentle manner, Frank was a pastor at his local church. He would often pick me up and take me places when I was too tired to walk. In soothing tones he would chat to me, telling me how God loved me and was using me in Africa. It was impossible to put a price of what that meant to me. He also announced he intended marrying the love of his life, Esther. She was simply gorgeous and had the loveliest giggle, and sometimes when she got started laughing she couldn't stop. They had set an 'introduction day' date, traditionally when the woman introduces her intended to everyone in her family and the man pays the dowry.

Esther's dowry list was budgeted at over one million shillings (about A$750) and started with a cow and finished with a suitcase. Everyone (including his best friend and the church committee) assists paying the dowry. In a way it is the African version of a bridal registry, and so I paid for a goat. I also did my UACO bit and gave him and Esther some family planning advice.

Frank had been seconded along with the hospital ambulance during CHOGM, which was held at the best hotel in town for four days and nights. Apparently, although some other ambulances look very fancy they don't have anything like the insides of ours: oxygen, a bed you can lift out, a fire extinguisher and a strong engine. Although Frank had no medical training, that was not uncommon. In Uganda ambulances are basically only for transporting patients between hospitals, or from hospital to house in rural areas. Frank told me he had to wear a special uniform for the occasion, and to prove it he came to collect me one morning in the ambulance wearing it.

'Shall I put the siren on for you, Mama Jude?' he asked.

As much as I wanted him to, I said, 'Perhaps just when we get to the hospital.' It was an added bonus that UACO received a large financial payment for the hire during CHOGM.

Chapter Twenty-Four

I HAD BEEN IN Uganda less than a fortnight when Fred Wilson's arrival from Australia caused great excitement, especially for Edward, who finally met the man he had been corresponding with for years. Rose turned on a lovely lunch which began with Frank offering a moving welcoming prayer for Fred. He was then treated like royalty by everyone at the hospital and clinic. Bukenya and Fred particularly hit it off, which was lucky given the number of hours they then spent together discussing how best to record and present information for AusAID accurately and professionally. Fred was handed two shopping bags full of documents by Bukenya for auditing. It was delightful having Fred helping, and jobs that often had taken me weeks only took us a couple of days. Fred stayed with me at the hostel. Because he had been involved with UACO since 2001 he had seen all the photos and video and heard my stories so was prepared for what he saw around him. He was excited to personally experience what he had heard about, especially the walking clinics, which he enthused were what UACO was all about.

Edward had organised big signs reading 'UACO is an AusAID sponsored project', following the procurement manual to the letter. Everything purchased for more than 50,000 shillings was paid by cheque and for any expenditures over a million shillings he got three quotes and tried for the best quality. Mosquito nets had gone up in price since we put in the application so were only able to buy about 600 instead of 950.

When not busy with the books, Fred was introduced to Ugandan-style worship. The first service we went to featured twenty minutes of uplifting choral singing followed by a sermon based on Romans 12, where Paul writes of the practicalities of love: *Rejoice with those who rejoice; mourn with those who mourn. Live in harmony with one another.*

Along with the reminder of spirituality came the reality of the cheapness of life. We heard news of a boarding school eight kilometres out of Kampala where a dormitory caught fire and girls were locked in. The power had gone off and it was believed the blaze began with charcoal or candles lit for light. More than twenty died. Edward's son Kenneth used to go there and it is recognised as one of the best schools in Uganda, having been set up by the king in the 1800s. Edward was truly distressed and grieving; his friend is the headmaster and often brought sick children to the hospital for treatment.

The small loans had mostly been used to start piggeries or cafés to date, but new ideas were springing up. One widow rented a tiny space under a shop verandah across the road from the hospital where she set up an alterations business. With a treadle sewing machine squeezed into her working area of about one square metre, sometimes she made clothes and hung them on the fence for sale but mostly she did mending. Before I left Australia, a woman from my church in Port Elliot, Sue Smith, celebrated her sixtieth birthday. Instead of spending money on a party, Sue said she wanted to make a difference for another woman in need and proposed buying a sewing machine and perhaps providing lessons for someone in Uganda. When I mentioned this to Edward and Persis they burst out laughing: before I arrived they had been talking about expanding the functional literacy class by having sewing machines and the like.

With Sue's donation plus a donation from one of Iva Quarisa's friends in Griffith we bought three treadle sewing machines, while UACO paid for a folding table to cut fabric on plus scissors, pins and needles. The students from all walks of life supplied their own material and thread and paid a small amount toward the teacher's salary. It evolved there were three tailors among the HIV/AIDS group so they were hired to teach the others. This truly put the 'function' into functional adult literacy, which was very exciting.

While some of those who received loans acted cautiously, others showed an entrepreneurial zeal. One was Ruth, who had been part of UACO since its inception and was the first secretary of the widows group. Her small mud brick house was one street back from a very busy road, and she used her loan to have the water put on. She had a stand pipe with a lock on it and sold water to her neighbours; Ugandans are often so poor that a basic thing like running water is a luxury. Ruth would deliver buckets or containers of water for a small fee. With her profits she extended her house and began renting a room out, then she bought a cow and was keen to add chickens. Her long-term plan was to move the cow to the rural village she came from, knock down what is now her cowshed and build a house to rent out (in Uganda a house often consists of just one or two rooms). She also had about five square metres of land which the widows wanted to rent to build a shelter for storing a truckload of charcoal, which they would sell off in smaller amounts. With the help of the extra money she had been earning, Ruth had been paying for her children's education. Two had now graduated from university and had jobs.

It was such a joy to see Bosco fit and well and working at his business. I was elated when he hugged me. What a colossal miracle from when I first found him bed-bound with pus pouring from infected sinuses in his legs, a urinary catheter draining into a bucket, unable to stand or do anything for himself. Then there seemed no hope of a better life, but now he moved freely and had a job cooking and selling food. In a bitter twist, someone stole his three charcoal cooking pots so he was reduced to cooking at home with a wooden fire. Despite this, he looked happy and well and had plans to expand his business by taking out a bigger loan.

Another individual donation from home had played a part in developing the micro-loan scheme. Viv Maskill from Melbourne, who had visited Uganda a few years before, sent money earmarked for the widows' education. We used the money for some infrastructure and a training day, organising a trip to the Katende Harambe Rural Urban Training Centre. This gave everyone a course in poultry, animal husbandry, horticulture, tree planting, animal fodder and biogas production. The information included specifics such as using cassava juice to make cement for house bricks, how to save water and using human and animal waste to generate methane gas for electricity.

Inspired, we organised a demonstration project for keeping chickens. The HIV/AIDS group put in the equivalent of $1.50 each which, combined with my donated money from Veronica Cullen of Victor Harbour, bought fifty day-old chicks. They were raised and sold at seven weeks old. There is a huge market for poultry in the street markets of Kampala, where chicks are bought by farmers who have larger farms and can run hens. This project was remarkable because it brought the HIV/AIDS group together to become responsible for raising the chickens. They all contributed a little money towards the cost of establishing it and then all took turns in caring for the chicks and repaying the loan. Some became so proficient that they applied for an individual loan to set up their own chick-raising business.

I found the work days exhausting. Every night I was weary but struggled to sleep and my Parkinson's was on the increase as a result of the stress and sleep deprivation. Iva had arrived two weeks after Fred and it was wonderful having them with me, and I wasn't the only one who appreciated their company. Paul Latolo from the youth group said that as I was called Mama Jude, Fred should be *Taata* Fred, meaning father. Fred had a huge smile on his face all day.

Clinic mornings were always busy. The mothers and babies started arriving before 9.30 and the line was still long at 1.30 pm. Fred helped give out jumpers he had brought with him which disappeared in no time. Many asked for a bigger size, which was a wonderful confirmation that the babies were healthy and fat.

The HIV/AIDS support group members all introduced themselves to Fred by individually stating that they were HIV-positive. They were eager for projects they could do as a group, such as learning how to make cakes and ribbon decorations, important for special events in Uganda (for example, the man at an introduction or wedding wears a huge artificial ribbon flower in his buttonhole).

A keen photographer, Fred brought his video camera to record the day-to-day work of UACO. He gave a running commentary of what was going on and we were later able to distribute it on DVD to supporters in Australia.

But even the best camera work in the world won't fully convey the plight suffered by some Ugandans. On a walking clinic we found a *jaja* living in a tiny, dark, airless room. To get to her we had to straddle a large drain that ran next to her place. There had been no rain for some time and very hot days, so the smell of rotting rubbish in the drain combined with the airless heat in her tiny room was oppressive. She had cut her foot quite badly and required a tetanus shot plus treatment at the hospital.

Iva and Fred worked very hard, but we managed to slip away from UACO duties for a weekend safari and to fulfil a dream of seeing the great animals of Africa. We joined a tour group headed for the Queen Elizabeth National Park. Although the bus seated nine, there was only the driver/guide, Paul, and an Englishwoman named Suzannah Richmond on board. Suzannah and her husband both worked for the British High Commission in Ethiopia, and she was on safari while he was on assignment in Moscow. She was delightful company and had lived a fascinating life. Paul was twenty-seven years old and had an encyclopaedic knowledge of animals, birds and the country. He was very gentle, respectful and professional.

We drove 420 kilometres west of Kampala through lush green country. Out the window we saw the poverty of regional Uganda. The mud houses were often crumbling and children were dressed in rags that only just covered their bellies enlarged by malnutrition. Some children were walking to school in the rain with banana leaves over their heads – the African umbrella. We drove near the western border of Uganda and Congo to Fort Portal and then south to the park and our destination, Mweya Lodge.

The weekend was a blend of relaxation followed by periods of high excitement in the bush. We had lunch on a huge verandah overlooking the Kazinga Channel, a forty-kilometre stretch of water linking Lake George and Lake Edward. As we ate, buffalo and hippopotamuses wandered into the water, followed by a huge bull elephant that threw dirt over his body and then went into the water for a drink. I was so excited that I think everyone around me was a bit amused. Eventually the whole family arrived and we had eight elephants – I was in heaven.

At night in the lodge you could hear the sound of the animals, like a quiet, rumbling motorbike. When I got up and looked out of my bedroom window, two huge hippos were grazing just near the door to my room. They apparently come by each night, which explains the armed guards around the lodge.

On both mornings we were woken at six and had a quick coffee before heading out. It was the most glorious time as we watched the sun come up, the early morning mist drifting on the channel and the animals suddenly appearing. There were waterbuck, hyena, buffalo, hippopotamuses, Ugandan kob, antelope and hundreds of birds. My favourite was the spoonbill stork because of its brilliant long red, black and yellow beak, which looks as though it has been hand-painted.

On the way back from our last tour, like an encore to a virtuoso performance, we passed an enormous elephant so close to the road I could have leant out the window and touched him. He was slowly munching through some purple flowers and looked up and flapped his ears as if to confirm what we all thought: I am so beautiful.

A couple of days after the safari we were again back on the roads of rural Uganda, but this time to distribute the birthing kits supplied by Zonta. We drove two hours west of Kampala on dreadful tracks, with Edward and Frank in front and Fred, Iva and me cramped in the back.

At the first clinic at Kiganda we were met by a delightful Catholic nun named Sister Bernadette. She excitedly showed us around the tiny St Matia Mulumba Hospital and clinic. As we nibbled on roasted peanuts, Sister Bernadette gave us a wish list of needs including a new vehicle and extra buildings. Edward made a truly lovely response, gently explaining what we do and how we came to be delivering the Zonta birthing kits. In rural areas of Uganda such as this, most births occur at home, usually without the help of a trained midwife and certainly without a doctor, so the delivery is often assisted by a community worker or friend. The genius of the birthing kits is the way they help overcome basic hygiene problems. After the kits were handed over, Iva presented Sister Bernadette with children's dresses and baby clothes she had brought from Australia.

The local medical officer, Dr Lawrence, joined us so now six of us were jammed in the car, with Edward sitting next to me and poor Iva squashed into the small seats in the far back. I had never been on such bad roads. We couldn't go any faster than twenty kilometres an hour and were tossed from side to side as the vehicle crawled deep into the Ugandan countryside. People were living in very simple, old and often falling-down mud huts. The children all seemed to be dressed in rags. Many called out *mzungu* as we passed.

When we finally arrived at the second clinic we were met by another nun and a nurse. Again there were requests, this time for a vehicle, new beds and the completion of a new children's ward, which had been started. I was shocked when we visited the tiny hospital to find a young man with dysentery in a bed alongside a small child in another bed with severe malaria. There seemed to be no infection control measures in place.

From the day I arrived back in Uganda there had been plans to celebrate the AusAID grant. Eventually, when Fred and Iva had both arrived and after much preparation, the grand day was upon us and the celebration began at the clinic at 10, where two enormous marquees had been decorated with balloons, streamers and flowers. Edward rounded up the younger members of UACO and anyone else with the energy to walk, instructing them to go out and tell Kampala what the Australian Government had done for them. He mapped out a four kilometre walk from the hospital gates along the main Entebbe road and back. A marching band fired up and Edward grabbed my hand declaring, 'We are going to lead them off!' The band, followed by Edward and me and then a group of UACO youths and HIV/AIDs victims, proudly marched out of the compound and into the streets. It was part-pride demonstration, part-circus as the band competed with the traffic and police escort. Fred was standing up in Edward's car and leaning out of the sunroof filming everyone as they marched. People waved and clapped from the footpaths as the parade continued down Entebbe Road, the main thoroughfare south of Kampala. It slowed one lane of traffic to a crawl and even held up the vice-president's car for a while (lovely!). The march eventually covered about four kilometres before circling back into the compound and returning to the clinic for the formalities.

Iva and I wore our *gomez* dresses, which everyone loved. Rose helped to select the material for them – electric blue for me and hot pink for Iva – while Persis had given us the undergarment to wear to make our dresses sit properly, essentially a cotton half-slip with a frill that sticks out around your middle. It made us look as though we had gained about ten kilograms overnight. One of the beautiful widows came up and enthused, 'Mama Jude, you look so beautiful and you have hips.' Fred wore a *kunzu*, the formal attire for Ugandan men, and everyone felt he had paid them a high honour.

Our next challenge was to sing the Australian national anthem, with Persis joining Fred, Iva and me after just twenty-four hours to learn it. She did very well, too, and we received a boisterous reception from the audience. That was followed by items from the HIV/AIDS group, singing from the dance/drama group, poetry from the widows group and speech upon speech upon speech from anyone who was anyone. They were all glowing in their appreciation of what UACO is doing and has done.

I had to make a speech, of course, but found Edward had planned to say most of what I had to say so I reverted to explaining the original proposal to AusAID – that it was our desire to empower the people of Uganda. This money from Australia was to improve health, wellbeing and future prospects, particularly for women and those with HIV/AIDS and malaria. I spoke of how learning could increase through literacy, professional development and small loans to reduce poverty and bring hope for the babies, children and youths of Najjanankumbi and Uganda as a whole.

After the speeches we handed out mosquito nets and bags of food to UACO members and refugees from Congo and Eritrea. Anyone who accessed services through UACO is required to become a member by registering their personal details and having a photo taken. In the past some people who weren't in need had come and sponged off UACO and this new system meant those in need received help. My sister-in-law, Margaret Beaumont, had made environmentally friendly bags for the volunteers who had contributed so much to UACO, which we'd filled with more than five kilograms of food each. They were ecstatic and started to dance as I went to present them, so naturally I danced towards them too. It was a true celebration of the worth of these wonderful people and their value to UACO.

The only disappointment of the day was the local newspaper's coverage of the event, reporting it as a political stunt by the politician who was present. There was no mention at all of AusAID and we were referred to as the Uganda Austria Christian Outreach. Edward and I went to see the editor to politely point out the errors, who suggested I purchase space in the newspaper to advertise my organisation. Instead I asked how he thought the Australian Government would feel when I told them Uganda cannot even print the right name of the donor country. He agreed to send his features editor to do a story of the work of UACO.

Fred had been in Uganda for nearly a month and as his time came to an end we called a final meeting. Everyone took the opportunity to farewell him in loving terms, but none more so than Bukenya – I will never forget the way he spoke of how much Fred had taught him and how he will always be in his mind and his heart. Fred and I both found the words moving and unforgettable.

As we put Fred on the plane we welcomed Anthony Catanzariti, a friend of Iva's from Sydney. Anthony is a secondary school teacher and had just returned from walking the Kokoda Track with a group of students. He soon had another group of young people following him when Iva and Anthony came with me on a walking clinic; it seemed every child in Najjanankumbi was calling out and following us.

On the clinic we delivered mosquito nets to the elderly and vulnerable and visited a dear little boy called Sendagire. When UACO workers first found the eleven-year-old he could not walk and so crawled everywhere. He had hydrocephalus, caused by an abnormal increase of fluid in parts of the brain which in children causes the head to enlarge. I had dealt with a lot of children with this condition during my six months at the Adelaide Women's and Children's Hospital, which was part of my original nursing training at the Royal Adelaide Hospital in the 1960s. The children were always captivating and made my heart melt. With frequent monitoring and treatment from Daniel, he was now walking on his thin little legs. Despite the progress I was afraid he would not live for long.

I couldn't get Sendagire out of my head and eventually went to Edward and Persis to plan how UACO could give him the best life possible. We developed a plan for the nurse, Daniel, to continue seeing him each week, monitor the size of his head and ensure he had food that was high in protein and carbohydrates. On top of his hydrocephalus he also had sickle cell anaemia and needed iron supplements, special feeding and pain-relieving medication. We found out his father was dead and his mother drank heavily; when I asked her what his name was she couldn't remember. Iva and I bought him some new trousers, a shirt and a pair of thongs. He was really precious and easily made his way into our hearts. We found out later from his brother that his name was Peter

Despite how hard Edward worked, he would always think to enquire how I was. I reminded him at times to rest a bit but he just laughed. On this visit he called me Judy almost all the time, only reverting to 'madame' or *Nambatya* every now and then. I had been worried that when Fred came I would cease to exist as when Allan visited, but not so. We truly had come to understand and appreciate each other.

Our plans for UACO were growing as always, this time thanks to the new grant. AusAID funding cannot be used for salaries but the extra money meant we were able to divert UACO funds to employ Daniel five days per week. In addition, Edward gave the program a second nurse to cope with the number of babies being brought in for immunisation. The nurse was paid by UACO for the hours she worked at the clinic and by Edward when she was back at the hospital. Then we employed Grace Luwalo as a counsellor for all the right reasons, including his pushy personality. He was forthright in dealing with people and I believed this would help make things happen rather than waiting for something to go wrong, as so often occurred in Africa. We increased the number of literacy lessons each week by three, so Paul's salary went up with the extra workload.

One day I visited Nakulabye to see Alice Zalawango at the Florence Nightingale Clinic. She was very excited to see me, despite being in the middle of 'renovations'. It was in the most awful, awful state, with one room cordoned off doubling as a treatment area and a delivery room with just a mattress on the floor.

I returned a week later with Iva and Anthony, because I wanted them to meet Alice and experience the horrors of the Nakulabye slums. Alice met us all dressed up in her *gomez*. She took us on a tour of the slums, which were as appalling as I remembered. During the tour, women began approaching wanting me to sponsor their kids, supply them with mosquito nets and do something about the abysmal state of their drains.

That night I couldn't sleep wondering if UACO could expand into Nakulabye. Alice had almost begged me to help, but history told me I couldn't work with her. However, my first two years in Uganda were with her – it was my apprenticeship. She has a good heart for her people and she taught me much. In the end I spoke with Edward about the dreadful situation in Nakulabye, and we decided to assist with primary health care education and some birthing kits. We discussed whether Daniel could go there in a teaching or advisory position. I asked Alice to contact Edward and follow up the offers but she didn't.

As our time in Africa began to come to end, there was time for celebrating and dancing. We had long planned to have a party for the youths because they had never had a specific celebration for themselves before. I waited until Iva and Anthony were there because they were younger and had more energy than I did and I knew just how much they were loved and appreciated by the youth group. More than eighty members attended. After speeches we handed out new UACO t-shirts and posed for an enormous group photo. The youth drama group played the drums and danced brilliantly for forty-five minutes without a break until the perspiration poured off them. The youths served lunch of beef, cabbage, Irish potatoes, thin spaghetti, a variety of fresh vegetables finely cut as salad, and a beautiful spicy vegetable relish. Then it was time to dance. Everyone joined in, from the *mzungus* to a tiny eighteen-month-old dressed in rags. It seems everyone in Africa is born with rhythm.

Next came the day of Pauline and Johnson's wedding. For probably the first and last time in our lives, Iva, Anthony and I were driven to a wedding in an ambulance. Edward's car was being used as a wedding car so it was the only vehicle left to take us.

The bride looked gorgeous, accompanied by eight bridesmaids and three little flower girls with little boy attendants. Johnson looked thin and ill from AIDS but stood proudly alongside his best man and two young attendants. The wedding ceremony lasted about an hour before we drove back to the clinic for a party.

When the bride and groom arrived they were met with the UACO drums and dancers and the brass band we had on the AusAID celebration day. Everyone stood up and waved white hankies (or, in my unprepared situation, a white tissue). I was asked to make a speech and discovered that I was actually standing in for the mother of the bride as both of her parents were dead. Pauline and her husband came and knelt in front of Edward and me and presented us with their cake before doing the same to the father of the groom.

There were lots of speeches, dancing and musical items. Paul, the literacy teacher, was in his element as MC, keeping the crowd in stitches with his jokes. Next came the gift-giving and I sat next to Edward while the others were presenting their gifts. He said this was what I had given them – the spirit of UACO. It was a very poignant moment for me when I thought of what

UACO had become and how close after the first visit I came to never returning.

Then it was time for the bride and groom to dance together, Pauline now in her gorgeous sparkly red dress. After a few minutes they came over and asked us to join them – Edward with Pauline and me with Johnson. We danced African style and soon everyone was on their feet again, clapping and dancing and laughing in celebration.

Chapter Twenty-Five

ON MY FINAL WALKING clinic we saw some really sad situations. One *jaja* named Veronica was in so much pain that Daniel went back for the ambulance to take her to the hospital. Her only son was badly ill with malaria, so one of the youths agreed to take care of her in the hospital. Another lady was living in the most awful bedroom. It stank, and the reason was because she was sharing it with bats. The youth group later returned in numbers to clean her house and agreed to make it a monthly appointment.

The night before flying home, I lay in bed while my mind swirled back over the past nine weeks. There had been noticeable changes in Uganda since my last visit. Some roads were better and it was cleaner, but traffic snarls dogged every journey. There was a lot of crime and violence associated with robberies, and children were abused in many heartbreaking ways. There is so much injustice there. It seems the rich get richer and the poor get poorer, same as anywhere.

But one thing I was sure of was that I was a richer person for being here. The final church service I went to on my last Sunday in Kampala was so powerful. The choir had me in tears long before they finished, while the last hymn was sung over and over, as if in private worship. The gospel reading was from Matthew:

Now when he saw the crowds, he went up on a mountainside and sat down. His disciples came to him, and he began to teach them saying: 'Blessed are the poor in spirit, for theirs is the kingdom of heaven. Blessed are those who mourn, for they will be comforted. Blessed are the meek, for they will inherit the earth. Blessed are those who hunger and thirst for righteousness, for they will be filled.'

I feel the power of God very strongly every day in Uganda. It is one of the most wonderful things about being there.

Regeneration and renewal was physical as well as spiritual. Overnight, two mamas gave birth. I took photos of them and one baby was almost pure white. It is a curious but common thing that babies in Uganda are born white and then darken over their first few days of life. One was so pretty, with wide alert eyes and a beautiful little mouth.

The children had brought me to Uganda and they continued to sustain me. Little Judy is growing up tall, thin and gorgeous. I taught her 'See you later alligator – in a while crocodile', which would be a cue for her to collapse into gales of laughter. I just love her to bits. Each day at lunchtime I would swing her around and give her a peck on the cheek which she returned.

Michele collected me at the hostel one evening for some Aussie food and company, and I was surprised and thrilled to see Suzan with her. She had grown quite tall and was now going to the Heywards' school. She was having ongoing minor surgery in Kampala to release her keloid scarring to enable her to stand up straight. Hopefully one day she will be able to have full surgery so she can lead a more normal life.

Beth's sponsorship had been taken over by others and it was lovely to see her while visiting Frank and Michele. She had grown tall and willowy and was still at school, but wasn't progressing. The plan was to try to protect her from unemployment and prostitution by keeping her at school as long as possible. She speaks English very well, is conscientious and can work in the house and cook meals, so I expect she will eventually find employment as a house girl.

Before I left I went to Nakulabye to see Thomas. I bought him his first pair of long trousers and long-sleeved shirt, and he agreed they were 'very fine indeed'. His mama manages a little stall selling vegetables and dried fish. Although she doesn't understand English, we managed to communicate somehow. Thomas is getting taller and Alice says he is a nice boy, although every time she sees him he is grubby. School is not easy for him because of a learning difficulty, and it's compounded by having no way of reading or writing when he comes home from school. Where he lives there is no quiet room, chair, desk or electricity. I hope he can learn enough to be able to get paid work when he is older. For now he is healthy and happy and surprisingly quiet when he is at school, considering the cheeky and boisterous three-year-old he was when we first met.

There are so many heartbreaking stories and so much need, but sometimes I had to stop and remind myself that by the end of that year we expected to immunise 5000 children at the clinic for free. As well as that, their mamas can get education, health care and the chance to build a small business from a micro-loan and climb out of poverty.

During one of our conversations, Edward shared his desire for the hospital and UACO to be merged into one entity. He dreams of the Busabala Road Hospital expanding its services to include an operating theatre, and when that is done to rename it and include UACO in the title. As part of his long-term plan he wants a percentage of any profits to be put into UACO so it becomes self-sustainable. One reason for uniting the two operations was to help ensure his own children would develop a heart for helping the poor, and to preserve the continuity of both the hospital and UACO if he should die tomorrow.

There was a lot of good in what he said, but I was also concerned about the future management given that most of us on the Australian committee were getting older; I myself was now sixty-five. For the first time I started thinking seriously about who might look after UACO in the future.

Chapter Twenty-Six

SEVERAL MONTHS AFTER RETURNING to Australia I received an email from Persis saying thirty-one members of the functional adult literacy (FAL) class had graduated at a ceremony organised by the Kampala City Council. It sounded like a typical Ugandan affair with plenty of speeches. UACO teacher Paul Lutalo was awarded a prize as the best FAL teacher in the district and won a scholarship to study at Makerere University. At the end of the formalities, the UACO students presented a poem written by another student, Rwomushana James, entitled 'FAL – our hope, our future'.

> Oh FAL
> The mother of civilisation
> The second chance giver
> The builder of hope
> In you we survive

Our future in your hands
Reading or writing
English you command
Hygiene you teach
The clean environment
Families we plan

Oh what joy you bring

Happy are our families
Which are functional
Because of FAL
FAL, you're the man
Lucky is he
Lucky is she
Who has FAL
The future is bright

If we needed any confirmation of how bright the future was, it came while collating information for a second application to AusAID. I was overwhelmed when I saw on paper what had been achieved in a single year: more than 4000 patients given free treatment, more than 7000 immunisations, and reduced incidents of malaria thanks to 600 treated mosquito nets. There were now eighty-six registered members of the HIV/AIDS club who received counselling, food supplements and medical care. The decreased mortality rate of those with the disease amazed us – it had been three years since the last client died.

But there was even more than that. The walking clinic had expanded from five to eight zones, visiting almost seventy people at least once per month unless a change in their medical condition warranted more regular visits. There were seventy-eight students in the FAL class and another twenty on the waiting list. The youth group had almost fifty members who met on weekends and school holidays. Although the impact of the group is harder to measure, anecdotally it is making a difference through the reduction in crime and the spreading of good health messages. They also volunteer for walking clinics. The small loan scheme is only limited by the availability of funds; there is a waiting list of people wanting loans. The people we have helped have been able to change their lives, feed their children, pay their school fees and have an income, however small. They now have health care and hope for the future.

It is a decade since I first stepped off the plane in Kampala on what I thought would be my one and only visit to Africa. I didn't think I had much to offer because I hadn't been a clinical nurse for thirteen years. My ability was in administration, though I always thought I had a degree in getting things done. I am so sure that if I had any idea what lay ahead I would never have even gone the first time. But God's plans for me have often been surprising, almost sneaky. Here I am a decade later and I wouldn't have missed one moment.

So where to from here? Edward has specialist doctors begging him to build an operating theatre for them to use. If that happens then those registered as members of UACO will continue to receive free treatment, including surgery, physiotherapy and rehabilitation. This is my dream and the focus for the next stage of my life. If we can raise $350,000 we can have that theatre. I am convinced it will happen.

The people who have impacted on UACO and my life are mostly still heavily involved. The first chairman of the youth group, Ronnie, did pay off his loan and is now married. Bosco continues from strength to strength and is now managing his life and his income. Although Godfrey will always struggle with his disability, I love him dearly and admire his courage and spirit – no-one lights up a room with a smile like him. Persis continues to manage the outreach in her calm, professional and gentle way; I cherish her love and friendship. Daniel is setting new goals for UACO in the community and everyone looks to him for care and advice.

Edward and Rose are my Ugandan family. Without an almost chance meeting with Edward on my first visit, I am sure I wouldn't have returned. Their love and care for me over the years has enabled me to achieve what I have. I think I am finally getting to the time of my life when I have to stop and consider the needs of my family as well as my own health. I can't ever imagine not being involved with UACO but I do know in the coming years it will be time to hand over the reins.

For some time I felt that Iva was the ideal person to take over. We think alike on so many matters, plus she has a heart for Uganda and its people and wants to make a difference. When we were together in Busabala in 2008 I posed the question, and she agreed to take on the role one day – neither of us knows when that day will be. What I want her to do until then is be my shadow on the next trip to see how she finds it.

I have watched Iva grow from a quiet, slightly nervous person on her first visit into a woman of courage. I know that she can make the hard decisions. This is tempered with gentleness that Ugandans have come to love. She once said to me, 'I might be too soft.' I smiled at her. 'You'll learn. I did!'

Acknowledgements

BEFORE FIRST VISITING UGANDA I had been planning my retirement, and one idle dream was to learn how to smock so I could make dresses for my granddaughters. When putting this book together I asked my daughter, Fiona, for a title suggestion, and she came back without a second thought: 'So much for smocking!' Although the title didn't make it, in the process of writing I have become intensely aware of how many people either directly or indirectly have been involved.

Reverend Dr Gillies Ambler, my spiritual guide and dear friend, taught me how to reach out to God and understand this change in my life and my call to Uganda. Emeritus Professor Anthony Radford's wisdom and training prepared me for Africa.

The UACO committee in South Australia encouraged and supported me, in particular Fred Wilson and his wife, Ailee. Fred has been treasurer from the start and I am sure he had no idea what this was going to involve. I have been overwhelmed at the constancy of love and support of the congregations of Port Elliot and Westbourne Park Uniting churches. The Quarisa family of Griffith became intricately involved in UACO and I will forever be grateful for their love and friendship.

Richard Hearn, CEO of Resthaven in South Australia, started me down the long road of collecting equipment for the hospital and clinic. The Kiwanis Club of Adelaide purchased and prepared the two containers which became UACO Central. The organisations and private donors who donated equipment for the various containers are too numerous to mention, but their generosity and assistance enabled the hospital to be completed and the clinic to function. The gift of an ambulance by St John Ambulance Australia SA Inc. is incalculable. The Australian Government through its international aid agency AusAID has allowed us to expand our services.

Thank you is such an inadequate reward for those who have donated money and continue to do so. You are the soul of UACO.

In Uganda, my thanks to Frank and Michele Heyward for their love and friendship and the opportunity to 'eat and speak' Australian from time to time. My dear friend Judy Howe from Canada shared her house, hopes, love and laughter with me.

I would have never seen the distance without the love and support of Dr Edward Ssembatya and his wife, Rose, my Ugandan family. Edward heads up a loyal and committed team in Uganda, in particular Persis, who manages the outreach, and Bukenya, the financial manager of the hospital and UACO. Without their loyalty and service UACO simply would not exist.

From the start of my journey to Uganda I have kept daily journals, not knowing one day they would become a book. It is completely due to Michael Sexton that this book has become a reality. Although many people in the past have said I should write it, I never considered it for a moment until Michael said he would like to have a go at a chapter. I treasure Michael's friendship, professionalism and expertise. I cannot thank him enough. The book was enthusiastically supported by Karen Penning at ABC Books and sensitively and constructively edited by Simone Ford.

Allan has always walked this journey with me and without him there would be no book at all. I would never have lasted the distance without his love, encouragement and reassurance.

Finally I must thank the precious people of Najjanankumbi for their acceptance of this *mzungu* who arrived in their midst, not knowing anything about them or their culture. I have been richly blessed by their love, teachings and friendship.

To find out more about UACO please go to our website

www.uaco.org.au

Our website contains lots of information about how we started, what we do and how you can support our work. There are also links to our newsletters and to reflections written by people who have visited us in Uganda.

If you don't have access to the internet, our contact details are:

Uganda Australia Christian Outreach
Westbourne Park Uniting Church
27 Sussex Terrace
HAWTHORN SA 5062

www.ingramcontent.com/pod-product-compliance
Lightning Source LLC
Chambersburg PA
CBHW022032290426
44109CB00014B/842